Jürgen Giessing

High Intensity Training

High Intensity Training

How to build muscles in minutes – fast, efficient, and healthy

by
Jürgen Giessing

ISBN-13: 978-1717452740

What this book is about

How many sets should be performed for optimal progress? How many repetitions per set for maximal muscle growth? How many training days per week are best? Which exercises are recommended? Split training or even double split training? How many warm-up sets? Heavy or light weight? Strict exercise form or cheating?

There are so many questions concerning training that it is not surprising that many people are confused. Looking at each of these questions may actually contribute to neglecting another question that is not only more important but also the base for all answers to these individual questions. And this question is:

How does training work?

Training processes have been studied for many years using the most recent scientific methods available. The relevance of training parameters (for muscle stimulation) as well as the importance of rest (for regeneration) have been identified in detail and provide us with all the information necessary to make the body adapt in the desired way to build up lean muscle.

This book is about how training works and what this means if the goal is to gain lean muscle. As a sports science professor I often come across misconceptions of training that have been disproved long ago but are still being passed on. One of these misleading concepts is the "the more, the better" approach that is still followed by millions of trainees world-wide. However, sports science has proven many times that the quality of training is much more important than its quantity. This book deals with the reasons for this "lie that will not die" and how current findings of sports science can be used to one's advantage.

Making the quality of training a priority has the pleasant "side-effect" that the quantity of workouts can be reduced. In fact, it even has to, if quality is the top priority.

If you want to know more about the theoretical background and practical implications for training, read on.

Table of Contents

What this book is about iii

1   Survival of *the fittest*? How much and what kind of
      exercise our body needs 11

2   How training works 23

3   Intensity of effort 39

4   The discovery of High Intensity Training 43

5   The (missing) scientific background of
      multiple-set training 53

6   The Holy Trinity: All good things come in threes 71

7   The paradigm shift that never happened 79

8   The essence of High Intensity Training 93

9   Training programs 107

      9.1   Sample full-body workout A 109
      9.2   Sample full-body workout B................................ 112
      9.3   Sample full-body workout C................................ 114
      9.4   Sample full body workout with pre-exhaustion A 116
      9.5   Sample full body workout with pre-exhaustion B 118
      9.6   Sample full body workout with post-exhaustion A......... 120
      9.7   Sample full body workout with post-exhaustion B......... 122
      9.8   Split program: Sample upper/lower body split.............. 124
      9.9   Split program: Sample upper/lower body split
          with pre-exhaustion 128
      9.10   Split program: Sample upper/lower body split
          with post-exhaustion...................................... 132

9.11   Split program: Push-pull split A (two-way split)............. 136

9.12   Split program: Push-pull split B (three-way split) 140

10   Intensity and consistency... 147

Recommended Reading... 149

Endnotes... 151

Acknowledgements.. 169

About the author 170

List of Figures

Figure 1:   Lack of physical exercise causes negative
             adaptation and regression.. 12
Figure 2:   Milo of Croton 21
Figure 3:   Improved muscle fiber activation precedes
             muscular hypertrophy 26
Figure 4:   The General Adaptation Syndrome (GAS) 32
Figure 5:   Friedrich Nietzsche... 33
Figure 6:   The process of supercompensation...................................... 34
Figure 7:   The training threshold 37
Figure 8:   Arthur Jones 44
Figure 9:   Cross referencing by physiologists who recommend
             the execution of multiple sets
             (Carpinelli, 2002, p. 320).. 55
Figure 10:   Strength gains after ten weeks of HIT compared
             to ten weeks of three-set training.. 59
Figure 11:   Mike Mentzer 83
Figure 12:   Drop set: reducing the resistance immediately
             after reaching muscular failure 99
Figure 13:   Leg press.. 109
Figure 14:   Back row 112
Figure 15:   Shrug.. 114
Figure 16:   Pec-deck fly.. 116
Figure 17:   Incline bench press 116
Figure 18:   Leg extension... 118
Figure 19:   Squat.. 118
Figure 20:   Lat pull-down... 120
Figure 21:   Pullover 120
Figure 22:   Dips 122
Figure 23:   Push-up... 122
Figure 24:   Leg curl... 124

Figure 25: Shoulder press...126
Figure 26: Leg extension...128
Figure 27: Leg press...128
Figure 28: Biceps curl...130
Figure 29: Leg curl...132
Figure 30: Calf raise..132
Figure 31: Dumbbell lateral raise..134
Figure 32: Chin-up 136
Figure 33: Incline dumbbell press...138
Figure 34: Back row 140
Figure 35: Abdominal crunch..142
Figure 36: Incline bench press 144

The images in Figure 1 and 2 were created by Udo Buffler. Julia Suchoroschenko created the image on the front cover, the images in Figure 3, 4, 6, and 7 and all portraits and illustrations of training exercises in this book (Fig. 5, Fig. 8, and Fig. 11-36).

List of Tables

Table 1: Intensity of effort: the four degrees.........................41
Table 2: Studies that found no significant difference in strength gains as a result of performing a greater number of sets (Carpinelli, 2002, p. 322) 60

1   Survival of *the fittest*? How much and what kind of exercise our body needs

For thousands of years adapting to the demands of one's environment and living conditions was the best one could do in order to survive. Those best suited to their environment and its particular demands on physical activity had the greatest chances of survival (and of passing on their genes). For thousands of years being the fittest meant being able-bodied and powerful. It meant coping with an environment by covering large distances every day looking for water and food, collecting whatever could be eaten, hunting and killing prey while avoiding being eaten at the same time. Therefore, those who were fast, strong and enduring were the fittest and had the best chances of surviving.

Today things are different. They have changed tremendously and are almost reversed. Those who best fit to their environment will not walk for miles each day. They are more likely to work in a factory or an office, carry a notebook instead of a spear and a meal-to-go instead of the prey they have hunted. They use contemporary methods of transportation like cars, taxis, planes, trains, busses, and the underground, which require almost zero physical activity from the passenger while travelling from one place to another. And this kind of modern, effortless transportation is not limited to roads and streets. It is also available within buildings. For example, there are elevators, escalators, assembly lines and other devices that transport items or people. Basically, hardly any physical activity is needed to be well-equipped for our modern world.

For the contemporary consumer food does not have to be picked from trees, much less hunted, killed and skinned. It is available in all kinds of variations from all around the world and in all seasons. Some kinds of food, especially fast food, are available 365 days a year 24/7 and can be ordered by a mouse click (which is physical activity, too, but not exactly intense) or a phone call and are delivered to our door step if we wish so. Instead of having to follow our prey for miles to finally hunt it down with intense effort, all we have to do is get up from the armchair and walk to the front door where we receive the ready-to-eat food. In terms of physical activity we have come a long way (or rather just the opposite) from what our ancestors had to do in order to survive.

The consequences of these changed living conditions are obvious. Unless we provide for it ourselves, we are tremendously lacking physical activity and, even worse, we lack resistance. Our muscles atrophy when there is no need for them to contract against an appropriate resistance. And this is a rational thing for the body to do. Why waste a lot of energy on maintaining resources like muscles when they are not needed?

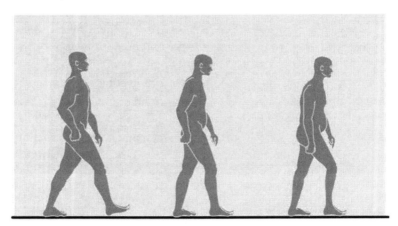

Figure 1: Lack of physical exercise causes negative adaptation and regression

In our modern world we are deprived of two things we desperately need in order to be healthy: physical activity in general and intense muscular contractions in particular. And we must clearly understand that the two are not the same: There is a difference between low-intensity aerobic activities like walking or jogging and intense anaerobic work like resistance training. Physically, our body benefits from both kinds of activity.

By simply increasing the amount of physical activity, like walking and running, we can improve our general well-being but it will not do much in terms of keeping our muscles from atrophying and keeping our bones dense. The solution to this problem is very simple. We have to do both. What we need is physical activity on a regular, preferably daily basis and regular workouts with a proper degree of intensity to stimulate muscle growth or at least keep our muscles from atrophying.

The World Health Organization recommends walking at least 10,000 steps per day for maintaining or improving health. It needs to be said that even though this is a reasonable rule of thumb, this number was chosen arbitrarily. Today, most people walk 5,000 and 6,000 steps per day on average whereas just a century ago our ancestors were likely to walk between 10,000 and 20,000 steps on an ordinary working day (which was basically every day).

Increasing our daily walking range is very simple. All we need to do is take the stairs instead of the elevator, park our car further from the office entrance, or leave the car in the garage when our destination is within walking distance. It is well documented that even small increases in physical activity will have a positive effect on health. And generally speaking: the more physical activity, the better.

However, and this needs to be pointed out very clearly, this "the more, the better" approach *cannot* be applied to muscle training.

However widespread this misconception may be, modern science has proven repeatedly that training stimuli need to be specific in terms of intensity, volume, duration, and frequency. To be effective, training has to be prescribed like medicine.

The more, the better?

The concept of "the more, the better" may be true for some things but it is definitely not a universal principle. This means that whereas it is beneficial to be physically active every day and get our 10,000 steps daily, working out every day is not necessary and may even be counterproductive.

Training volume, i.e. the quantity of training, is just one aspect of a complex process that consists of at least four interdependent factors: intensity, volume, duration, and frequency.

There is a prevalent but inappropriate overemphasize on the *quantity* of training (volume, duration and frequency) whereas the importance of *quality* of training (intensity of effort and perfect form) is often underestimated.

Volume, duration and frequency are thought to be the crucial factors for best training results because it seems to be logical that the more you train, the better results you will get out of your training. But that is not the case. There is no proportional correlation at all between the time spent training and the extent of physical improvement.

This misconception arises when transferring facts from one context to another. But *working out* is not the same as *working* even though both terms contain the same verb. In fact, *working out* is completely different from working in many ways. If someone has a job and is paid a certain amount of money per hour, then there is a proportional correlation between the time spent working and the amount of money earned. The more you work, the more money you get. Therefore, it may seem natural to suggest applying the same approach to working out.

Falsely assuming that there is a proportional correlation between training volume and training results, however, is to miss the whole point of training.

Intensity, rather than volume, is the crucial factor that decides whether a successful training stimulus can be achieved. If training is not intense enough, there will not be any need for the body to adapt. This is a well-known fact that is often overlooked.

Too much volume may compromise intensity and thereby compromise the effect of the training session altogether. Intensity and volume are inversely proportional. Training can either be intense or long, for example running can either be a long-distance run or a sprint but not both. There is no such thing as a sprint marathon. The same applies to resistance training. The more intensely you work out, the sooner you will fatigue. You can either train intensely or you can train long.

Therefore, training programs should be planned by determining adequate training intensity first, that is a degree of training intensity to surely pass the training threshold. Then all other factors should be adjusted accordingly.

Many people still believe that there is a proportional correlation between training quantity and training results, although they are not likely to not get better results the more they work out. Many people spend hours upon hours in the gym every week, yet they are disappointed with their progress. So why do they not question the concept of "the more the better"? This is no surprise considering what psychologists call *effort justification*.

Effort justification

Whenever we realize that the results we get out of something clearly do not match the amount of work we put into it, we find ourselves in a state called *cognitive dissonance*. In order to relieve ourselves from that unpleasant condition we tend to justify the effort and try to convince ourselves that "it is/was all worth it". This is one reason why things that we have worked a lot on are more valuable to us. Someone who buys an old-timer and spends hundreds of hours working on it is unlikely to sell it a few years later, even if offered much more money than the purchase price.

If you went to dozens of garage sales until you found that out-of-print book which you had been looking for so long, how likely are you to sell it later? If someone studies at a University for years to pass the final exam and get the degree, it will be extremely valuable to that person, even if he or she chooses a completely different career option later for which the degree would not have been necessary.

The Sistine Ceiling paintings by Michelangelo are among the world's most famous and most admired pieces of art. The fact that it took Michelangelo from 1508 to 1512 to finish his paintings illustrates what an effort it took to create such an outstanding piece of art. It makes us appreciate it even more.

Art is only one example where effort justification can be found. There are many others. Even architecture is one of them. The pyramids of Giza are a wonderful example of this. Although there are many higher and larger buildings today, the pyramids of Giza remain to be outstanding and rightfully remain one the Seven World Wonders. After all, it took presumably 20 years of incredibly hard work to build them and they remained the tallest man-made structures in the world for more than 3,800 years. It is very unlikely that four thousand years from now the same will be said about some of the buildings from the 20th century.

In 1929 Thomas Mann was awarded the Nobel Prize in Literature, mainly for his splendid novel *The Buddenbrooks* which consisted of 768 pages. On the other hand, the 1954 Nobel Prize of Literature went to Ernest Hemmingway for his great short-stories and his grandiose 99-page novel *The Old Man and the Sea*.

The bottom line is: We might have every reason to value the effort that somebody puts into something, but whenever actions are taken to achieve a certain result, the key issue always is how adequate these actions are to achieve that particular goal.

More about Nobel Prize winners: In 1905 Albert Einstein finished several publications. All of them were so ingenious that the year 1905 was later called the *wonder year of physics*. One of these publications was Einstein's doctoral thesis. When Albert Einstein first handed in his PhD thesis to Professor Alfred Kleiner, his doctoral advisor, Kleiner felt it was brilliant, yet he initially hesitated to accept the dissertation. The *only* thing that Kleiner criticized was that he felt Einstein's dissertation was "zu kurz" (German for "too short") for a doctoral thesis. It consisted of 17 pages.

A scientist may spend his or her whole life trying to solve a problem or might solve it through a sudden flash of inspiration. Some of the greatest discoveries or inventions were brought about by coincidence. Alexander Flemming (another Nobel Prize laureate) discovered the substance he later called Penicillin when returning to his laboratory after spending some weeks on holiday with his family. When he came back he found one culture of staphylococci contaminated with fungus which destroyed the staphylococci near the fungus. His further research finally led to the development of the world's first antibiotic.

This discovery was responsible for millions of lives that could be saved by fighting serious infections with antibiotics.

But should we value Flemming's work less because of the fact that the breakthrough in his research happened accidentally? I do not think so. Should Einstein have added some meaningless pages to his already brilliant piece of work? What if Michelangelo had not needed five years to finish his Sistine Ceiling paintings? What if he had finished them within six months? Should this make us appreciate his work less – or even more?

A side-effect of effort justification is that we do not only appreciate something more if we had to spend a lot of time on getting there. We also tend to attribute this success to the amount of work that we spent and underestimate the relevance of the quality of the process. After all, it is the result that counts, not the amount of hours we spend to get there.

We are rightfully impressed when someone says: "My car broke down. I called the mechanic who did not give up until he finally found the mistake after nine hours and then fixed it." But is it not equally admirable if the story goes like this: "My car broke down. I called the mechanic who took one look at it, found the mistake and fixed it on the spot." In the first version our appreciation for the mechanic's effort is most likely caused by his not giving up, his persistence to keep looking for the mistake, but not his quality as a mechanic whereas in the second version the competence and efficiency of the mechanic clearly stand out.

Achieving the same result in much shorter time by improving the quality rather than the quantity of effort, improves the efficiency of the whole process tremendously.

Efficiency and the time factor

Everybody knows the saying "time is money" (usually attributed to Benjamin Franklin). However, this statement is incorrect. In fact, time is much more valuable than money. According to psychologists Philip Zimbardo and John Boyd time is our most valuable possession. And who could argue with that.

With regard to classical economics Zimbardo and Boyd point out that the rarer a resource is, the greater is its value. Unlike most other things that can be possessed like jewelry, gold or money, time cannot be replenished. Their statement that "(...) nothing will allow us to regain time misspent" [1] hits the nail on its head.

The outstanding value of time is also reflected economically. Overnight delivery is more valuable because of the time saved and therefore more expensive than regular delivery which may take a few days. International flights are another example. Non-stop flights are more expensive than connecting flights with a stopover that may even require a change of planes before reaching the actual destination. Although connecting flights (sometimes called "direct" flights to hide the fact that it is not a non-stop flight) cause higher costs for the airlines, they can charge more for non-stop flights because they help us save our most valuable possession: time.

Training is no exception. A training program is more efficient if it produces the same results or even better results in less time. And that is why High Intensity Training is the most efficient kind of training there is.

Those who say "I don't care if I am wasting a lot of time in the gym as long as I am making good progress" should think twice. Even if there was no such thing as overtraining, which in fact impairs training progress, there is another factor that nobody can escape from: *opportunity costs*. This is another economical principle that also applies to time. And since time is our most valuable possession, it even applies more to time than to anything else.

Just as money spent on one thing cannot be spent on something else, the time we spend in the gym cannot be spent doing something else. Even if somebody does not mind wasting time in the gym (over)training, opportunity costs of that decision cannot be denied.

And there is one opportunity cost directly related to too much time spent training: Every minute spent (over)training means less recovery time from the workout. So training more than necessary is not just a waste of time. It is much worse than that. Training more than necessary (regardless of whether the person may enjoy time spent training) is counterproductive!

For this reason it is obvious that the "the more, the better" concept neither makes sense in an economical nor in a physiological context. Actually, the principles that are responsible for making muscles bigger and stronger have been identified a long time ago and could have been available for more than two millennia.

Recently, training science has rediscovered the legend of Milo of Croton which illustrates how the process of muscle training works in a nutshell. The lessons that can be learned from this famous ancient legend have been ignored for too long.

Milo of Croton

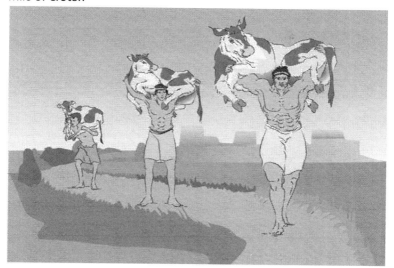

Figure 2: Milo of Croton

Milo of Croton was an Olympic wrestler who lived in the 6th century BC. In fact, he may have been the most successful wrestler in Olympic history. He won the wrestling competition at the ancient Olympic games several times and was also a multiple winner of the wrestling competition at the Pythian Games at Delphi. Milo remained unbeaten for about a quarter of a century. Contemporary authors described Milo as incredibly strong. Milo, a friend of ancient mathematician and philosopher Pythagoras, allegedly once saved Pythagoras from being crushed when the roof of the house they were in broke down. Milo supported the central pillar until Pythagoras and the others could get out and then he saved himself by rushing out.

Unlike other strong men in history who were described as "naturally strong" or "blessed by God with outstanding strength" young Milo was the opposite. He was a very weak child and was beaten by the kids in the neighborhood more than once. But Milo was determined to do something about that.

According to the legend, Milo took a baby calf, put it on his shoulders and carried it around his parents' farm. He did that exercise once every day. After several years the calf had grown to a full-grown bull so that eventually Milo was carrying a bull around the farm. Not only had the baby calf grown but so had Milo's strength. His muscles had developed due to the progressively increasing training stimulus that they were exposed to on a regular basis.

The legend of Milo may be a bit exaggerated but it clearly shows some of the constituent parts of how training works. Obviously, among other elements, training must be:

Intense enough: It took a lot of effort and strain to lift and then carry the bull. Carrying a mouse would not have made Milo the strongest man of his time.

Progressive: Lifting the same weight in every workout will neither stimulate muscle growth nor strength.

Regular but infrequent: After working out the body needs time to recover from the strain of the workout. After adequate rest and recuperation (and time for positive adaptation), the next workout can follow. Working out once in a blue moon will not be enough to cause any positive adaptation.

Apparently, this knowledge has been available for more than two thousand years.

By the way: How many "sets" of bull-carrying did Milo perform during each "workout"? That's right – just one!

2   How training works

Although all the important components of training have been contained in the story of how Milo became so incredibly strong and muscular, it took more than two thousand years before the components could be properly identified. As a consequence, many misconceptions about training have developed. Some of them are still around today.

Maybe the biggest misconception is applying the idea of "the more, the better" to training. Training is like medicine. You need a certain dose. Once you reach the required dose, the medicine will cause a physiological reaction. Taking more than the required dose is not necessary. In fact, it is even counterproductive and even potentially harmful. This is why every medicine comes with a package insert that informs and warns you of the dangers of an overdose of that medication.

So where does this misconception of more training being better come from? This question can be answered quite easily. In many contexts it is absolutely correct that the more you do the better you become. If you want to be the best piano player you can be, you better play a lot. Playing the piano only twice a week for twenty minutes will not do much to improve your ability of playing the instrument well. This concept even applies to some aspects of competitive sports, at least to a certain extent.

It is true that there are many kinds of sport in which potential success is directly related to the numbers of hours spent. Many competitive athletes follow a high-volume approach when preparing for important sports competitions or even the Olympics and World Championships.

In some sports this is absolutely reasonable because preparation for competitions on an elite level consists of two factors:

a) practice

and

b) training.

Practice

When it comes to practicing tactics, moves, games and so forth, the old saying that "practice makes perfect" is definitely true. If your goal is to hit the basket as often as possible, many hours of practice will help you improve more than practicing just a little bit once in a while. If you are the quarterback of a football team, you would do well to practice all the passes and tactics and everything that is needed to be successful. Soccer players spend a lot of time not only practicing the basics like ball control. They also need to practice set pieces like corner kicks, free kicks and so forth, not only to improve their own skills but to learn how to play together successfully as a team. After all these hours of practicing they usually know what a certain teammate will do in the next moment. They know where he will run and where the ball must be passed in order to be received by the teammate.

Even in power sports like weightlifting, practice is a very important factor. The more often you practice a certain movement, the more skillful your movement's execution becomes and eventually you will reach a level of execution that can hardly be improved even further. Thus, practicing improves performance in many sports. Improvements by practice result from improved skills, experience and coordination. Up to a certain point it is very likely that the more you practice, the better you will become. However, practicing should always cease before exhaustion sets in. No gymnast with exhausted leg muscles would practice their routine on a balance beam and no table tennis player would try practice his serve when feeling exhausted. Throwing the darts can even become quite dangerous to yourself and others once you have lost your concentration and your arms start to shiver due to the amount of throwing that has just been done.

Once you have perfected your technical skills, more practice will not generate better results. A high jumper who already uses perfect form on the Fosbury flop cannot improve his high jump by practicing more often. But stronger legs will enable him to jump higher. And that can only be achieved by *training* them. Although both terms are often falsely considered synonyms, training is a completely different process.

Practice must precede training

Training must be preceded by successful practice. Take the bench press for example: To gain muscle strength by performing bench presses, the proper execution of that exercise (or any exercise for that matter) must first be mastered. When this is the case, it still takes several workouts before increases in muscle mass can be expected. This may come as a surprise to many trainees who have experienced strength increases right from the start of their training program. And indeed, the greatest increases in strength occur during the first half year of training. This seems to contradict the fact that it takes several weeks of training before muscles grow but there is a very logical explanation. When the body is confronted with a previously unfamiliar stimulus it reacts first by recruiting more muscle fibers for which there has so far not been any necessity to contract. Then, as the training process continues for weeks, more muscle fibers are recruited, which results in increased strength. Once the maximum number of muscle fibers that can be activated voluntarily has been reached and the training program is continued, the only way muscle strength can be increased even further is by hypertrophy in the trained muscle fibers.

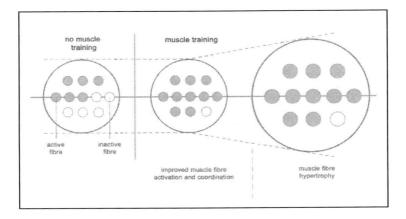

Figure 3: Improved muscle fiber activation precedes muscular hypertrophy

Training

Muscle hypertrophy is never the result of practice, it can only result from physiological adaptations.

If an organism is confronted with a stimulus that surpasses a certain threshold level, it will adapt to that stimulus. If you are trying to get a sun tan and expose your skin to a certain level of ultraviolet radiation for a certain amount of time, it will adapt by increasing pigmentation. Once that reaction has been triggered, further exposition to the same stimulus does not add to the effect. In fact it may even reverse the effect by burning your skin so that the tan is lost again.

If your dentist gives you an anesthetic injection which successfully frees you from your pain, a second or third injection will not give you an additional advantage. Giving you dozens of injections may even kill you.

Whenever the human organism is confronted with a certain stimulus above the threshold level the corresponding reaction is triggered. Muscle training is no exception. If a muscle is confronted with a certain amount of tension (about 50-80% of max) for a certain amount of time (about 60 to 120 seconds), the muscle goes into hypertrophy and gains mass and strength.

Stimulus-reaction scheme and ceiling effect

This is called the stimulus-reaction scheme and does not only apply to muscle training but to all kinds of adaptations of the human body to external and internal stimuli. There are two interesting facts about the stimulus-reaction principle and the ceiling effect:

a) Once the reaction has been triggered, it cannot be stopped anymore.

b) Once the threshold has been surpassed, adding stimuli does not fortify the effect.

This is shown by the previous example of the dentist giving a local anesthetic for the nerves of a painful tooth:

a) Once the required amount of medicine numbs the nerve, the process can no longer be stopped and you will be free of pain.

b) Giving you another injection will not make you feel "even more free of pain".

This also applies to the process of immunization. After a successful vaccination you are immune to the respective illness. Another injection two minutes later will not make you "even more immune".

Neither will a third one another two minutes later. The principle of stimulus-reaction scheme applies to any physiological adaptation. Pregnancy is caused by one single sperm successfully fertilizing the ovum. Additional sperm also reaching the ovum will not make you "more pregnant".

Probably one of the reasons why High Intensity Training is so popular among medical doctors is that they know about the *stimulus-reaction scheme* and are familiar with the *ceiling effect*.

The ceiling effect describes the fact that once the stimulus reaction has been triggered, further stimuli will not add to the effect. If you need 200 milligrams of a certain medication to reach its maximum effect, raising the dose to 300 or even 400 milligrams will not make the medication "work even better". Actually, the opposite is true. The more unnecessary medication somebody takes, the more side effects are likely to occur, eventually doing more harm than good.

The same applies to training. Once you were successful in stimulating hypertrophy in the trained muscles, the muscles need rest to let the growth process take place. Adding more stimuli (more sets) will not initiate more hypertrophy. It might even interfere with recuperation and, thus, be counterproductive.

Basically, the misconception of more training being better is a transmission error caused by applying a perception to *training* that has been derived from observations of *practice* ("the more, the better"). However, such a transfer is inappropriate and unduly.

People who watch a high jumper practice his jumping in the stadium might attribute the strength and size of his leg muscles to his many hours of practicing. What they usually fail to see is that those muscles were not built by practice. They were built in the gym – by training them intensely.

Most people are not aware of this necessary distinction between practice and training and they cannot be blamed for that. Even many exercise professionals and experts have only recently come to realize how important a clear distinction between practice and training is. This lack of differentiation that has been around for centuries is also reflected semantically. Most languages did not even have a word for *training* and adopted the English word. The word *exercise* stems from the Latin word *exercitium* which for centuries has been translated into *practice*. In German, an exercise is still called *Übung*, which literally means *practice*. However, those exercises will only result in physiological adaptations if they are performed with an appropriate degree of intensity followed by enough rest for the body to recuperate and adapt to the stimulus.

In a nutshell, this is how training works. As simple as this may sound, it took the legend of Milo and more than two thousand years for this insight to become generally accepted. At the beginning of the 20th century athletes still had to go by trial and error in order to find out what worked for them and what did not. However, even if their exercising resulted in improvements, they still did not know what exactly caused these improvements. Was it the kind of exercises? Was it the number of training days per week? The order of exercises? The amount of weight or resistance used? The number of sets per exercise? The number of sets per workout? The rest time between sets? The number of repetitions per set? The speed of each repetition? These are only a few questions about training. Obviously, there are many more and, in addition to that, there are just as many questions concerning the role of nutrition, rest, sleep and so forth. Whenever an athlete made progress, something was obviously working. But it was not known exactly *what* was working and *why*.

As a consequence of this lack of knowledge, aspiring athletes did something very understandable. They copied the whole daily routines of successful champions. They copied not only their training routines but also their eating and sleeping habits.

Despite the fact that all the necessary information on training is available to everybody today, many people still do what their ancestors did more than 100 years ago. They copy the training routines of the "champs" and end up training six to twelve times a week like an Olympic athlete, hoping that doing the exact same routine as the champ will put them into the exact same shape as the champ, ignoring genetic factors (not to mention drugs) and not realizing that

a) most of the training articles that are printed in the magazines are grossly exaggerated in order to make the story more interesting and to sell unnecessary food supplements

b) a rather large amount of the "training" time of professional athletes consists of practicing what they need to do in order to perform well on the day of their contest

Understanding physiology

In the 19th century the German toxicologist Hugo Schulz discovered that the growth of yeast was reduced by large amounts of poison (no surprise here) but was actually *stimulated* by a small dose of poison. This observation caused some surprise among the scientific community but was then largely ignored for several decades.

During the 1930s two very important observations were published that showed that this principle also applies to human physiology. In an article that appeared in the scientific journal *Nature* Hans Selye, a medical doctor explained his observation that there are three different stages in which the human body reacts to "noxious agents", which he later called "stress".

The other important finding was published in the book *The Wisdom of the Body* by Walter B. Cannon. Inspired by the works of French physiologist Claude Bernard, he explained that the human body has a tendency to keep up a state called homeostasis (a kind of equilibrium with relatively constant conditions of energy levels, temperature, pH hydration etc).

Small changes do not disturb homeostasis because the body is able to regulate itself. If a person has a daily energy demand of, for example, 2000 kcal, this person will not gain weight when consuming 2050 kcal nor lose weight on 1950 kcal a day. The body can regulate energy expenditure up or down a few percent to keep everything balanced. But if homeostasis is disturbed more severely, a physiological reaction is inevitable.

Selye's book *The Stress of Life* (published in 1956 and later translated into 17 languages) explained for the first time that a stimulus is needed which exceeds a certain threshold level to have an impact on homeostasis. When this homeostatic balance is disturbed by any stimulus, the body reacts by trying to adapt to it. Selye also found out that this reaction consists of three different stages: the alarm reaction, the stage of resistance and the stage of exhaustion. Since the body's reaction to stress can be generalized, Selye called this process the General Adaptation Syndrome (GAS).

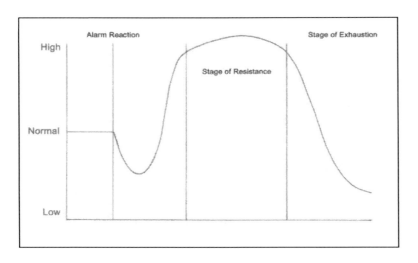

Figure 4: The General Adaptation Syndrome (GAS)

Überkompensation

Another observation in this context is the fact that overcoming an illness or disease usually makes the organism stronger and thus less susceptible for future illness. As the German philosopher Friedrich Nietzsche had already written more than a century earlier:

"What does not kill me makes me stronger" ("Was mich nicht umbringt, macht mich stärker").

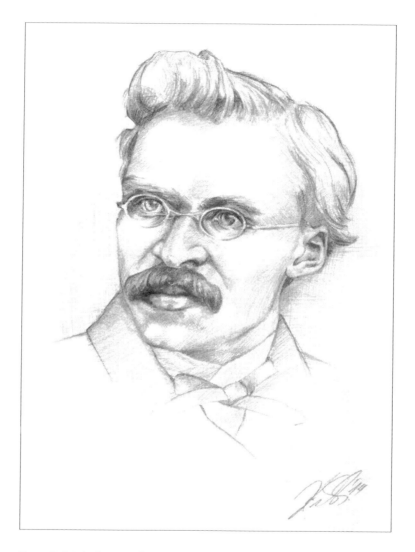

Figure 5: Friedrich Nietzsche

In the 1970s scientists discovered that this adaptation mechanism not only applies to the body's ability to cope with illness but also to any kind of other stressor, including physical exercise.

It was discovered that once the body has recovered successfully from a stimulus, it not only restores the previous status quo but surpasses that point to better cope with future stress that might even be more intense. The process was first described by the Hungarian scientist Nicolai Jakowlew in 1976 pointing out that the body does not only compensate the effects of the particular stressor(s) but goes beyond this by *over*compensating to protect the body from negative consequences of the same kind of stressor in the future. German scientists called this *Überkompensation*. Another synonym is *overcompensation*, whereas Jakowlew preferred the Latin term *supercompensation*.

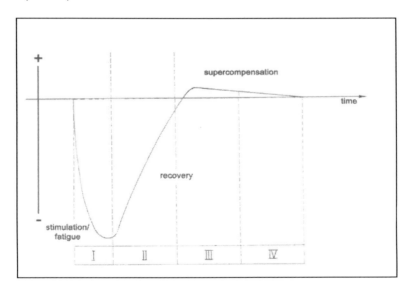

Figure 6: The process of supercompensation

The graph that demonstrates the process of supercompensation does not go with a time frame. That is because different actions take place in the body as a consequence of a training effect. These different actions do not all happen at the same time. Body temperature and hydration, for example, are regulated within minutes after training. Energy balance can also be restored rather quickly but other processes like muscular adaptations take days and adaptations of tendons and bones take even longer.

We know from medical contexts that once a stimulus surpasses a certain threshold, the corresponding reaction is triggered. If the body is then given time to rest, it will adapt to that stimulus in a functional way. Further applications of the same stimulus before the body has adapted, will not add to the effect and might even interfere with the body's ability to adapt to the stimulus. This is the reason why one sufficiently intense set of each exercise is all that is needed to stimulate muscle gains. The trained muscle fibers then do not need more sets of the same exercise. What they rather need is enough time to rest and grow.

Recently, the model of supercompensation gained a lot of attention. The brilliant scholar and bestselling author Nassim Taleb uses the model to explain his concept of *antifragility* and points out that there is a lesson to be learned from the body's ability to supercompensate that can be transferred to other contexts as well. Taleb points out that supercompensation is a natural mechanism of the body to "fight the next war" by overcoming the last one and preparing for the next one. This is how resistance training makes us stronger: *"(...) the body overshoots in response to exposures and overprepares (up to the point of biological limit, of course)."* [2]

There is no doubt that intensity is the key factor for an increase in strength and muscle mass, not volume. Milo lifted a progressively heavier bull once every day. Lifting and carrying a baby calf twelve times a day would not have made him as strong and muscular. Observations in occupational medicine have shown the same. Intensity, rather than the volume of activities is responsible for physiological adaptations.

Imagine somebody working in an office or book shop from 9 to 5 sorting letters into different filing systems or putting books on different shelves (or a similar kind of work). Lifting 100,000 letters, each weighing 100 grams, adds up to a total workload of ten tons or 10,000 kilograms. Despite the impressive volume of 100,000 repetitions and 10 tons of weight, this kind of "exercise" may eventually give you sore shoulder joints or arthritis but will do nothing in terms of strength and muscle building. On the other hand, lifting 100 kilograms ten times with maximum effort will be more effective for muscle building, despite a total workload of only 1,000 kilograms.

The bottom line is: There is a training threshold. If this training threshold is surpassed, a training stimulus is created. If the threshold is not surpassed, there is no need for the body to adapt. This can be illustrated by another example from the mail delivery business. There are mailmen who walk from door to door for six to eight hours each day, which easily adds up to a walking distance of 40 to 70 miles a week. How many mailmen do you know who can do well in, or even win, a 10,000 meter race without any specific kind of training? Considering the volume of their physical activities, one might think they should easily be able to do that. But it is quite obvious that the intensity of walking is not sufficient to surpass the necessary training threshold. As long as they do not train, simply being active will not be sufficient, not even at a very high volume.

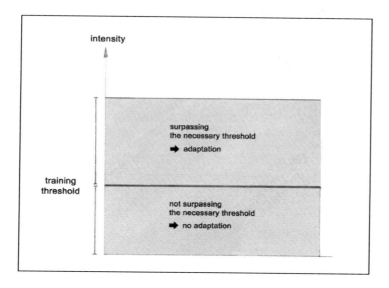

Figure 7: The training threshold

Again, it should be noted that this fact is not limited to muscle training but applies to any aspect of the body adapting as a result of imposed demands.

On a dark and cloudy November day you can spend all day sitting on your veranda without getting a tan. The intensity of sunshine is not high enough to surpass the threshold that is needed for the body to adapt. On a hot and sunny summer day, however, ten to forty minutes of unprotected exposure to the ultraviolet radiation of the sun will stimulate pigmentation in most people. Extended exposure time will not result in a deeper tan but in sunburn.

It is impossible to calculate exactly how many minutes in the sun are needed to get a tan (like X minutes of exposure to Y electronvolt at a wavelength of Z) but it is safe to say that you better get out of the sun when your skin is starting to look a bit reddish.

3 Intensity of effort

The same applies to training intensity. We do not know (and most likely will *never* know) the exact point when the threshold is exceeded. Fortunately, it is not necessary to know. What we do know is that high intensity training ensures a sufficient training intensity level to trigger adaptations in terms of strength and muscle hypertrophy. Therefore the important question is not "Am I doing enough sets?" but rather "Am I training intensely enough?".

And there is an answer to that question. Again, the calculation is the same as in other physiological contexts. If you need a particular medication, your doctor will calculate how much you need based on your age, sex, body weight and other factors. If your doctor's calculation comes to the result that you need 186 milligrams a day, he will then tell you to take 200 milligrams a day to make sure you get enough but not too much of the required medication.

It is the same with training intensity. If you are able to do ten chin-ups in perfect form but fail on the eleventh repetition, you did the most you can do for that exercise. You may already have surpassed your individual training threshold during repetition number nine or ten, but finishing the tenth repetition and even trying to finish the eleventh makes sure the training threshold is exceeded. Therefore, it is safe to say that training intensity is the key factor for physiological adaptations.

Unfortunately, the term intensity is often misunderstood. It is necessary to distinguish between *relative intensity* and *training intensity (also called intensity of effort)*.

Relative intensity refers to the weight that is used for a certain exercise in relation to one's *one repetition maximum* (1RM). The 1RM is the maximum amount of weight that can be lifted once. If a lifter is able to lift 100 kg once, but not twice, and uses 60 kg for that particular training set, then this person is training with a relative intensity of 60%. If this person is not able to lift this weight more than twelve times in one set, then this weight represents the person's 12RM.

This may sound complicated. But the good news is that you do not have to worry about relative intensity. It has been proven many times that it does not matter if you chose, for example, 59%, 62% or 71.9876 % of your 1RM for your training set as long as you perform your exercises in proper form throughout the set, perform repetitions slowly and without unwanted momentum and "train to failure". In other words: Any resistance that will cause you to reach "muscular failure" within a time span of about 60 to 120 seconds is absolutely appropriate for triggering strength and muscle hypertrophy.

High Intensity Training is not about lifting very heavy weights. It is about maximum effort. As long as you train to muscular failure, it does not matter if you could have used 2% more weight but it does make a huge difference if you could have done two more repetitions instead of training to failure!

It is not surprising that there is a widespread misconception about High Intensity Training allegedly requiring super heavy weights because some people confuse *relative* intensity with intensity of effort. The term intensity referred to in the acronym HIT refers to intensity of effort which could also be described as the maximum effort that is necessary to perform a set to muscular failure.

Intensity of effort can be categorized into four different degrees:

Table 1: Intensity of effort: the four degrees

nRM	non repetition maximum Terminating a set at a fixed number of repetitions or a certain rate of perceived exertion whereas additional repetitions are possible.
RM	repetition maximum Terminating a set after the final repetition that can be completed in proper form.
PMF	point of momentary muscular failure Terminating a set when concentric failure has been reached, i.e. the final repetition cannot be fully completed due to fatigue.
PMF+	training beyond the point of momentary muscular failure Training beyond failure by applying high intensity training methods like forced repetitions or drop sets

Which degree of training intensity is necessary to surpass the necessary threshold for stimulating the corresponding adaptations? We still do not know whether it takes at least, for example, 95% of maximum effort or rather 97.23%. What we do know, however, is that performing a set at maximum effort will induce adaptations in terms of strength increases and muscular hypertrophy. Therefore, training sets should never be terminated before the repetition maximum (RM) has been reached.

Sometimes even that is not enough. Let's say you have just done nine good repetitions in perfect form and feel that you might not be able to complete another repetition. Well, there is only one way to find out whether you really cannot do another one. In other words: Only when you reach the point of momentary muscular failure during your, for example, eleventh repetition, you know for sure that ten repetitions were your 10RM for that set.

4 The discovery of High Intensity Training

"Intensity of effort is almost the entire answer in itself; lacking the proper intensity of effort, little or nothing in the way of results will be produced by any amount of exercise – At least not in the way of muscular size or strength increases. But given the proper intensity of effort, then very little in the way of exercise is required for the production of best possible results." [3]

The fact that it is intensity of effort rather than the volume of training that is responsible for physiological adaptations like strength and muscle gains was discovered by Arthur Jones. The term "discovered" probably describes it best, although it may seem inappropriate at first sight. However, it would be even more inappropriate to call it an "invention" since HIT is merely based on observations of how the human body reacts and adapts to high intensity stimulation of muscles.

Arthur Jones (November 22, 1926 – August 28, 2007) was born in Morilton, Arkansas and grew up in Seminole, Oklahoma. Coming from a family of medical doctors (including his mother and his father, one grandfather, his sister, his brother-in-law, his uncle and his cousin) Arthur Jones took an interest in human physiology from an early age, having read his parents' entire medical library as a boy. Without any doubt, he was a man with many talents. He was a pilot, a big game hunter, a producer of TV documentaries, an inventor, an entrepreneur, and a manufacturer of exercise machines. In his first publication (Nautilus Bulletin No. 1) Arthur Jones introduces himself as an airline pilot who has "conducted a large-scale import-export business in wild animals, birds, reptiles and tropical fish – an occupation which eventually led to the production of films based on conservation themes."

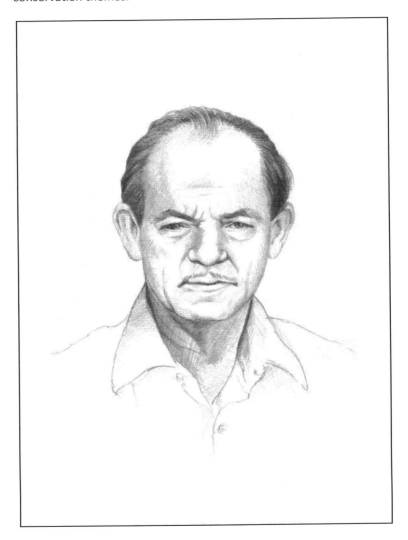

Figure 8: Arthur Jones

In fact, his documentary "wild cargo", was first broadcast in the United States in 1961, and became a great success on American TV like several of his other documentaries. Also, it was broadcast in several countries in Europe. One of Arthur Jones' observations during his years in the animal kingdom made him think twice about the intensity and volume of his own workouts. After studying wild animals for years he noticed that very muscular animals like the male gorilla or the male lion do not move much, but when they do, they hunt or fight with maximum effort and incredible intensity. Jones described the physical effort of a hunting or fighting lion as "very intense but infrequent". He figured that this kind of physical effort was an important factor for the outstanding muscularity of these animals [4]. It appeared logical to Jones to apply the same approach to his own training. And that is what Jones did. Previously he had been training very much, up to four hours a day, six or seven days a week. Now he cut back his training to three non-consecutive days per week, reduced the number of sets to 16 for each of his full-body workouts and made sure to take every set to momentary muscular failure.

This routine put him into the best shape of his life. Whereas the best condition he had previously achieved by doing a typical volume training had been a weight of 172 lbs/78 kg (at a height of 5'8/152 cm), his low-volume high intensity training got Jones into the best muscular condition of his life at 205 lbs/93 kg [5].

Jones went on coaching bodybuilders in using his High Intensity Training method and developing and selling exercise machines ("Nautilus") that earned him a fortune. The fact that Jones sold exercise equipment has often been (ab)used by his opponents to discredit High Intensity Training accusing Jones of promoting HIT just to sell his training equipment. However, Jones published several books and more than one hundred articles in which he explained how High Intensity Training works and always pointed out that High Intensity

Training can be done by using any kind of equipment and that it takes less than a dozen exercises to complete a full-body workout.

Jones' concept of High Intensity Training can be summed up as follows:

- Use proper form on all exercises and perform each repetition very carefully and slowly avoiding using momentum at all times.

- Perform one set per exercise, always training to muscular failure.

- Choose a moderate resistance that makes you reach muscular failure after about eight to twelve repetitions. If you can do more repetitions, increase the resistance for the next workout.

- Train twice a week (never less than once and never more than three times a week) allowing for proper rest between workouts for the body to recover and supercompensate.

- Train your whole body in every workout. Starting with the bigger muscles and progressing towards the smaller ones.

- Do not take drugs.

Basically, these recommendations contradicted everything that trainees were told at that time. In contrast to Jones' recommendations the type of training that was *en vogue* during the early 1970s called for multiple sets of each exercise ("the more, the better"), several exercises per "muscle group" ("the more, the better"), to split "muscle groups" by training them on different days, and to train each muscle group twice or three times each week ("the more, the better"). Training to failure, however, was usually not advised because it was supposed to be "dangerous". Another then established believe was that once a trainee progresses, the number of sets per exercise had to be increased, too. Therefore, single-set training, if it had any use at all, was thought to be suitable only for beginners whereas advanced trainees were advised to do two, and after progressing further, move up to the supposedly optimal training volume of three sets per exercise.

A widespread belief at that time was that single-set training, regardless of its intensity, was never enough to significantly increase strength or even muscle mass, especially not in experienced trainees. Jones, however, found the opposite to be true as a consequence of his own experience and started to train bodybuilders accordingly. Among them was Casey Viator who had first met Arthur Jones after the Mr. America contest in 1970 where Viator placed third. One year later, after training under Jones' tutelage, Casey Viator won the 1971 Mr. America contest at the age of 19, which made him the youngest Mr. America ever, a record that still stands today.

Viator's success with High Intensity Training and Arthur Jones's publications (Nautilus Bulletins No. 1 and No. 2) as well as his articles in publications like Iron Man Magazine, Athletic Journal, Muscle Training Illustrated, and Muscular Development received a lot of attention among athletes and especially among bodybuilders. Several professional athletes, many bodybuilders and some scientists visited Jones' Nautilus facility in Florida to find out more about High Intensity Training. Among them was Dr. Elliot Plese, director of the Exercise Physiology Laboratory at Colorado State University. What particularly caught Plese's attention was that trainees not only gained strength and muscle mass from High Intensity Training, as expected, but also improved their cardiovascular condition and flexibility, which was the exact opposite of what people at that time believed were the consequences of strength training.

Muscle training was thought to make people lose agility and speed and become "muscle-bound", slow and stiff. At that time, many scientists and medical doctors (among them the renowned Dr. Kenneth Cooper who coined the term "aerobics") advised people to participate in long-duration but low-intensity exercise while completely avoiding strength training. High intensity activities especially were considered to be dangerous. So the results of High Intensity Training that Dr. Plese witnessed at Jones' Nautilus facility were the exact opposite of what leading experts of that time were teaching. Plese was particularly impressed with the progress that Casey Viator had made.

In 1972 Jones and Plese came up with the idea of carrying out an experiment at Colorado State University to evaluate an individual's development in terms of increasing strength and muscle mass within one month. Initially, Jones had planned to conduct such an experiment at his Nautilus facilities in Florida, where he had everything he needed including access to all the training equipment he considered ideal for that purpose. However, Jones dismissed the idea when he realized that the authenticity of the outcome would be questioned if the whole experiment was not monitored by an independent supervisor. As Jones later wrote in his Nautilus Bulletin No.3, the expected outcome would run "directly contrary to widespread opinion". In that same publication Jones explained the aim of the planned experiment:

"Among other things, we hoped to demonstrate that (1) very brief workouts are capable of producing rapid and large scale increases in muscular mass and strength...(2) nothing apart from a reasonably balanced diet is required...(3) the so-called "growth drugs" are not required." [6]

Originally, Arthur Jones was intended to be the only subject in this experiment. Jones and Plese thought that as a successful competitive bodybuilder Casey Viator had already reached the peak of his potential and could hardly improve his condition even further. Arthur Jones on the other hand would make a much more "realistic" subject. He then was a man in his 40s who had been training on and off for several years and had found it hard to stick to a regular training program due to his impressive work schedule. The experiment was set to begin on May 1st in 1973 and end on May 29th, giving Jones exactly four weeks of training.

Four months before the experiment was scheduled to begin Casey Viator was injured in an on-the-job accident and lost part of a finger. An allergic reaction to a tetanus injection he received afterwards was so severe that Viator could not work out for four months. The four months of illness, not working out and eating far less than his usual diet resulted in a weight loss of almost 33 pounds (15 kilograms). In April 1973, when Casey Viator had recovered, he became a perfect candidate for the experiment to find out how much of his lost muscle mass he would be able to gain back during the four weeks of the experiment.

The Colorado experiment

The experiment started on May 1st 1973 as scheduled at the Exercise Physiology Laboratory at Colorado State University in Fort Collins, Colorado. The experiment was supervised by Dr. Eliot Plese. Body weight, fat-free mass and body fat were measured by Professor James E. Johnson using the Whole Body Counter in the University's Department of Radiology and Radiation Biology. Weighing and testing procedures were repeated on May 29th for Casey Viator and on May 26th for Arthur Jones.

Both subjects performed three training sessions per week, separated by at least 48 hours, consisting of a single set taken to the point of momentary muscular failure. Every workout consisted of ten exercises chosen from the following list of available exercises: leg press, leg extension, leg flexion, pullover, pulldown, neck press, rowing, hyperextension, biceps curl, triceps extension, parallel bar dips, supinated chin up, and standing press. Chin ups and dips were done using regular equipment (parallel dipping bars, chin up bar) whereas the rest of the exercises were executed on Nautilus machines created by Arthur Jones, some of which were still prototypes at that time. Both subjects were on a high-protein diet consisting of regular food and no food supplements.

Casey Viator worked out 14 times during those four weeks, training his whole body in each session (total training time 7 hours and 51 minutes), whereas Arthur Jones, for health reasons, could only train his upper body and worked out twelve times (total training time 4 hours and 48 minutes) during the experiment.

When the final tests were done, the results achieved were outstanding for both subjects. Arthur Jones had increased his lean mass by 20.1 pounds while losing 1.83 pounds of fat. Casey Viator's results were even more remarkable. He reduced his body fat by 17.93 pounds and gained 63.21 pounds of lean mass. His performance of the standing press increased from eight repetitions with 217 pounds to eleven repetitions with 287 pounds and his leg press strength increased from 32 repetitions with 400 pounds to 45 repetitions with 840 pounds. In the initial strength test Viator did twelve parallel bar dips with an additional 50-pound plate attached to a belt around his waist. In the final strength test Viator did 16 repetitions with an additional 100-pound plate.

As mentioned before, there was no doubt as to the accuracy of these strength increases and muscle gains since all the data was collected and recorded by members of the University of Colorado and several people were present to witness training sessions as well as the testing.

The before and after photos of Jones and Viator as well as a full report of the results were published in Iron Man Magazine and created quite a furor in bodybuilding and fitness circles.

Just as Jones had predicted, there was a consensus among those who had been pushing the "the more, the better" concept of training. They claimed that Casey Viator's achievements could be explained by his exceptional genetics or that he must have been taking anabolic steroids during the experiment (which Viator always denied). Other arguments were that he was *re*gaining mass, which is easier than building new mass and that Jones used the experiment to advertise his Nautilus training equipment. But all of these arguments, however true, are irrelevant because they miss the point of the experiment. The aim of the experiment was to demonstrate that one set of each exercise, taken to the point of momentary muscular failure two to three times a week, is all it takes to increase strength and muscle mass and that food supplements are not necessary if regular high-protein food is consumed in sufficient quantities. Although Casey Viator's results may indeed be far from what the average person can achieve, considering that he had exceptional genetics for the sport and had already been very successful as a competitive bodybuilder, the results achieved by Arthur Jones were indeed remarkable. And they were the result of high intensity single set training.

Unlike Viator, Arthur Jones was neither a competitive athlete nor a young man nor particularly gifted in terms of genetic potential for muscle growth. Despite the fact that he was not completely healthy during the experiment he was able to (re)gain 20 pounds of muscle by training only twelve times, working out less than a total of five hours. This was less than some the top bodybuilders at that time were training per day, and definitely a lot less training than most experts were recommending *per week*.

Proponents of high-volume training either ignored the results of the Colorado Experiment or dismissed it as being "propaganda" for high intensity training and claimed that one set per exercise was not enough training volume to result in improved strength and muscle mass, and science had proved that three sets of an exercise were the ideal number and far superior to single set training for building muscle. But when you actually take a good look at the scientific literature, none of these statements can be validated.

5   The (missing) scientific background of multiple-set training

For generations trainees have been told that the more they train, the better their results will be. As discussed earlier, this may indeed – to a certain extent – apply to practice, but definitely does not apply to training. Several studies have in fact shown that results will *not* improve significantly if multiple sets of an exercise are performed instead of one. So why do several authors – and many coaches – claim that science proves there is a proportional relationship between set volume and training results?

As incredible as this may sound, this whole misconception was caused by a single study published in 1962 that was completely misinterpreted and told people what they wanted to hear anyway.

More than half a century ago a study by Berger (1962) claimed that three sets of ten repetitions were best to increase strength in the bench press [7]. So three sets of ten repetitions became the standard training recommendation. However, when looking at the data published in the study (which not many people did) it became obvious that the differences between one set and three sets were only marginal and *statistically insignificant* for almost all combinations of sets and repetitions! Single-set training actually produced results comparable to three-set training. So instead of "three sets of an exercise are best", the results of Dr. Richard Berger's study should rather have been summed up as: *One set of an exercise produces results comparable to those of two-set training or three-set training.*

Another result of the Berger study was misunderstood as well. Berger's data clearly shows that one set of six repetitions produced *more* strength increases than two sets of six repetitions. However, these differences were also statistically insignificant. There were in fact no statistically significant differences between one, two and three sets of bench presses. This was simply ignored by many who have used the results of the Berger study to "prove" that three sets of an exercise will produce optimum results in strength training.

The Berger study was then used by several other authors as a reference for the superiority of multiple-set training over single-set training. An overview of this cross-referencing can be found in Dr. Ralph Carpinelli's superb article "Berger in retrospect" published in the British Journal of Sports Medicine [8]. In this overview Carpinelli lists 67 publications that recommend multiple-set training. The authors of these publications "prove" their recommendation by either referring to the Berger study itself or by referring to one of the several other publications, which again refer to the Berger study as the only "proof" for the "superiority" of multiple-set training:

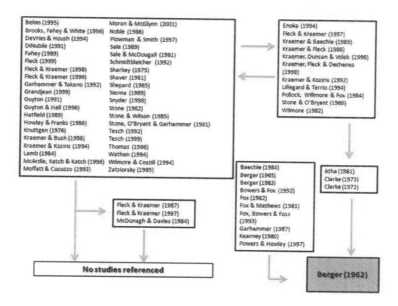

Figure 9: Cross referencing by physiologists who recommend the execution of multiple sets (Carpinelli, 2002, p. 320)

"Three sets are best": A myth is born – and is still passed on today

The Berger study seemed to have answered the question of how many sets per exercise are best and there appeared to be no need for additional studies. The cross-referencing of Berger's study in many articles not only spread the information among the strength training community but also created the impression that there were dozens of studies proving the superiority of three-set training. Three sets became the standard. Those 67 publications claiming three-set training as being ideal and offering scientific proof for this (all "proof" from by the same study) may have created the impression that there are 67 studies showing three-set training to be superior to single-set training, which obviously is not the case.

Not much attention was paid to the fact that for most repetition schemes Berger's study did actually *not* find statistically significant advantages for doing three sets rather than one set. It was also overlooked that Berger's results showed better improvements for one set than for two sets. Also important is the fact that intensity of effort was *not* properly taken into consideration at all in this study. Since Berger wanted to compare the effects of the number of sets and repetitions per set, each subject was told to perform an exact number of repetitions per set (e.g. "do three sets of ten repetitions"). Subjects then had to terminate the set once the designated number of repetitions had been reached, even if they could have done more repetitions [8]. When they could not perform the designated number of repetitions, they were assisted by a training partner to complete the given number of repetitions. This means that the intensity of effort was not controlled at all. Some subjects trained beyond the point of momentary muscular failure whereas others trained at a very low level of intensity and did not get near their actual repetition maximums. Subjects also rested between sets and exercises as much as they liked. Each of them performed additional exercises that were not reported in the publication of the study, including exercises that involve the same muscles as are used in the bench press like shoulders and triceps.

Later Berger conducted more studies comparing single-set and multiple-set training, all of which showed *no* significant differences between single-set training and multiple-set training. However, he still recommended doing at least three sets per exercises in all of his publications, citing his own study from 1962 as a reference [9-14].

Considering the limitations of the Berger study it is rather surprising that this single study was enough to seemingly provide the so-called scientific foundation for designing training programs for millions of people world-wide.

Additionally, not only the authors mentioned above recommended three-set training. Most of the "muscle magazines" picked up the information that three sets were believed to be ideal and spread the recommendation among their readers. One very vocal advocate of multiple-set training was Dr. Fred Hatfield. Hatfield was not only very successful as a powerlifter but also as a writer. He published several dozen books (including the book *Anabolic Steroids: What kind and how many*) and hundreds of articles in which, among other things, he promoted multiple-set training, and the use of supplements. In some of those articles Hatfield was very critical about High Intensity Training, always pointing out that science had proven the superiority of multiple-set training. On his website he wrote:

"Dr. Richard Berger (my mentor during my doctoral studies at Temple) years ago showed that there IS a significant improvement in gains with three sets as opposed to one. Other studies have shown the same results. Nowadays, many athletes (bodybuilders included) do as many as ten or more sets." [15]

This very interesting quote shows that Dr. Berger and his 1962 study influenced not only other scientists but also a man who would later become one of the most influential writers for the "muscle magazines."

Dr. Hatfield is definitely right by stating that "nowadays, many athletes (bodybuilders included) do as many as ten or more sets". There can be no doubt that some athletes do train with very high volume. For example, the former professional bodybuilder John DeFendis once even recommended doing up to 60 sets for each body part. But what does that prove? The fact that some do many sets does not mean that those sets are necessary.

Other bodybuilders were even more successful by doing only one very intense set per exercise. Examples are Mike Mentzer who won the Mr.

Universe title with a perfect score or Dorian Yates who won several Mr. Olympia titles. Dorian Yates trained very intensely but no more than three or four times per week. He regularly beat competitors who trained *twice each day*. Not to mention Casey Viator who became the youngest Mr. America winner ever by training only three times a week for 30 to 40 minutes and by doing only one set per exercise.

Years ago, when several meta-analyses were published which concluded that multiple-set training programs produced greater increases in strength than single-set programs [16-19], many experts felt that this was the final proof for the superiority of multiple-set training. The National Strength and Conditioning Association even announced "the end of the single-set versus multiple-set discussion." [20]

This conclusion may well have been somewhat premature. Meta-analyses are supposed to compare one particular aspect to another (in this case: single-set training to multiple-set training) *with all other variables being equivalent*. But in fact, if several studies are put together into one big meta-analysis, it is often questionable whether all other variables are indeed comparable.

In the case of the aforementioned meta-analyses studies were included that differed in several aspects, such as the subjects' age, sex, training experience, the kind of exercises used, the number of repetitions per set, the number of exercises used, the number of workouts per week, rest time between sets, rest time between workouts, study duration, and most importantly: intensity of effort.

Improvements in strength tests due to multiple-set training are often a few percent higher than those of single-set training when the subjects are beginners rather than experienced trainees. This is not at all surprising. Strength tests test not only strength itself but also to a large extent coordination, i.e. the skill of performing a given test exercise as well as possible. Performing and thereby practicing a certain lift three times in each training session will improve skills and coordination in beginners more than performing that lift only once.

A recent study showed that after ten weeks of HIT or three-set training subjects performed better in strength tests. However, body composition analysis revealed that more subjects who performed HIT gained muscle mass than subjects who performed the three-set training. But even those of the three-set group who did not gain muscle mass achieved better results in the strength test that followed the ten weeks of training than before the training program. The strength gains of those who did not gain muscle mass were obviously caused by improving coordination [21].

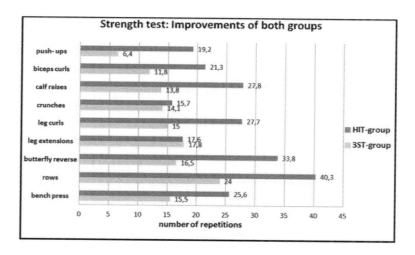

Figure 10: Strength gains after ten weeks of HIT compared to ten weeks of three-set training

After ten weeks of training, 71% of the subjects who performed HIT gained muscle mass compared to only 25% of the subjects who performed three-set training. HIT not only led to muscular hypertrophy in more subjects than three-set training, strength improvements were greater in the HIT group, too [21].

As we have seen, the Berger study and other publications supporting multiple-set training have received a lot of attention and have been quoted extensively. This cross-referencing and the attempt of the NSCA to put an end to the discussion of the necessary number of sets may create the impression of a consensus that multiple sets of an exercise were indeed necessary for optimum results.

Studies that show no difference between the two approaches, however, are often overlooked. In his article "Berger in retrospect" Carpinelli (2002, p. 322) lists the following *57 studies that found no significant difference in strength gains* as a result of performing a greater number of sets [22].

Table 2: Studies that found no significant difference in strength gains as a result of performing a greater number of sets
(Carpinelli, 2002, p. 322)

Number of sets	Studies in alphabetical order:
1 and 2	Capen, E. K. (1956). Study of four programs of heavy resistance exercise for development of muscular strength. *The Research Quarterly, 27,* 132-142.
	Coleman, A. E. (1977). Nautilus vs Universal Gym strength training in adult males. *American Corrective Therapy Journal, 31,* 103-107.
	Girouard, C. K. & Hurley, B. F. (1995). Does strength training inhibit gains in range of motion from flexibility training in older adults? *Medicine and Science in Sports and Exercise, 27,* 1444-

1449.

Graves, J. E., Holmes, B. L., Leggett, S. H., Carpenter, D. M. & Pollock, M. L. (1991). Single versus multiple set dynamic and isometric lumbar extension training. In *Eleventh International Congress of the World Confederation for Physical Therapy. Proceedings Book III* (pp. 1340-1342).

Hurley, B. F., Redmond, R. A., Pratley, R. E., Treuth, M. S., Rogers, M. A & Goldberg, A. P. (1995). Effects of strength training on muscle hypertrophy and muscle cell distribution in older men. *International Journal of Sports Medicine, 16*, 378-384.

Koffler, K. H., Menkes, A., Redmond, R. A., Whitehead, W. E., Pratley, R. E. & Hurley, B. F. (1992). Strength training accelerates gastrointestinal transit in middle-aged and older men. *Medicine and Science in Sports and Exercise, 24*, 415-419.

Lemmer, J. T., Ivey, F. M., Ryan, A. S., Martel, G. F., Hurlbut, D. E., Metter, J. E., Fozard, J. L., Fleg, J. L. & Hurley, B. F. (2001). Effect of strength training on resting metabolic rate and physical activity: age and gender comparisons. *Medicine and Science in Sports and Exercise, 33*, 532-541.

Martel, G. F., Horblut, D. E., Lott, M. E., et al. (1999). Strength training normalizes resting blood pressure in 65- to 73-year-old men and women with high normal blood pressure. *Journal of the American Geriatrics Society, 47*, 1215-1221.

Menkes, A., Mazel, S., Redmond, R. A., Koffler, K., Libanati, C. R., Gundberg, C. M., Zizic, T. M., Hagberg, J. M., Pratley, R. E. & Hurley, B. F.

(1993). Strength training increases regional bone mineral density and bone remodeling in middle-aged and older men. *Journal of Applied Physiology, 74*, 2478-2484.

Miller, J. P., Pratley, R. E., Goldberg, A. P., Gordon, P., Rubin, M., Treuth, M. S., Ryan, A. S. & Hurley, B. F. (1994). Strength training increases insulin action in healthy 50- to 65-year-old men. *Journal of Applied Physiology, 77*, 1122-1127.

Nicklas, B. J., Ryan, A. J., Treuth, M. M., Harman, S. M., Blackman, M. R., Hurley, B. F. & Rogers, M. A. (1995). Testosterone, growth hormone and IGF-I responses to acute and chronic resistive exercise in men aged 55-70 years. *International Journal of Sports Medicine, 16*, 445-450.

Parker, N. D., Hunter, G. R., Treuth, M. S., Kekes-Szabo, T., Kell, S. H., Weinsier, R. & White, M. (1996). Effects of strength training on cardiovascular responses during a submaximal walk and a weight-loaded walking test in older females. *Journal of Cardiopulmonary Rehabilitation, 16*, 56-62.

Pollock, M. H., Graves, J. E., Bamman, M. M., Leggett, S. H., Carpenter, D. M., Carr, C., Cirulli, J., Matkozich, J. & Fulton, M. (1993). Frequency and volume of resistance training: effect on cervical extension strength. *Archives of Physical Medicine and Rehabilitation, 74*, 1080-1086.

Pratley, R., Nicklas, B., Rubin, M., Miller, J., Smith, A., Smith, M., Hurley, B. & Goldberg, A. (1994). Strength training increases resting metabolic rate and norepinephrine levels in healthy 50-65-year old men. *Journal of Applied Physiology, 76*, 133-137.

Rhea, P. L., Ryan, A. S., Nicklas, B., Gordon, P. L.,

Tracy, B. L., Graham, W., Pratley, R. E., Goldbert, A. P. & Hurley, B. F. (1999). Effects of strength training with and without weight loss on lipoprotein-lipid levels in postmenopausal women. *Clinical Exercise Physiology, 1,* 138-144.

Rubin, M. A., Miller, J. P., Ryan, A. S., Treuth, M. S., Patterson, K. Y., Pratley, R. E., Hurley, B. F., Veillon, C., Moser-Veillon, P. B. & Anderson, R. A. (1998). Acute and chronic resistive exercise increase urinary chromium excretion in men as measured with an enriched chromium stable isotope. *Journal of Nutrition, 128,* 73-78.

Ryan, A. S., Treuth, M. S., Rubin, M. A., Miller, J. P., Nicklas, B. J., Landis, D. M., Pratley, R. E., Libanati, C. R., Gundberg, C. M. & Hurley, B. F. (1994). Effects of strength training on bone mineral density: Hormonal and bone turnover relationships. *Journal of Applied Physiology, 77,* 1678-1684.

Ryan, A. S., Pratley, R. E., Elahi, D. & Goldberg, A. P. (1995). Resistive training increases fat-free mass and maintains RMR despite weight loss in postmenopausal women. *Journal of Applied Physiology, 79,* 818-823.

Ryan, A. S., Pratley, R. E., Elahi, D. & Goldberg, A. P. (2000). Changes in plasma leptin and insulin action with resistive training in post-menopausal women. *International Journal of Obesity, 24,* 27-32.

Ryan, A. S., Hurlbut, D. E., Lott, M. E., Ivey, F. M., Fleg, J., Hurley, B.F. & Goldberg, A. P. (2001). Insulin action after resistive training in insulin resistant older men and women. *Journal of the American Geriatrics Society, 49,* 247-253.

Treuth, M. S., Ryan, A. S., Pratley, R. E, Rubin, M.

	A., Miller, J. P., Nicklas, B. J., Sorkin, J., Harman, S. M., Goldberg, A. P. & Hurley, B. F. (1994). Effects of strength training on total and regional body composition in older men. *Journal of Applied Physiology*, *77*, 614-620.
	Westcott, W. L. (1986). 4 key factors in building a strength program. *Scholastic Coach*, *55*, 104-105, 123.
1 and 3	Bemben, D. A., Fetters, N. L., Bemben, M. G., Nabavi, N. & Koh, E. T (2000). Musculoskeletal responses to high- and low-intensity resistance training in early postmenopausal women. *Medicine and Science in Sports and Exercise*, *32*, 1949-1957.
	Curto, M. A. & Fisher, M. M. (1999). The effect of single vs. multiple sets of resistance exercise on strength in trained males. *Medicine and Science in Sports and Exercise*, *31* (suppl), S114.
	De Hoyos, D. V., Herring, D., Garzarella, L., Werber, G., Brechue, W. F. & Pollock, M. L. (1997). Effect of strength training volume on the development of strength and power in adolescent tennis players. *Medicine and Science in Sports and Exercise*, *29* (suppl), S164.
	De Hoyos, D. V., Abe, T., Garzarella, L., Hass, C., Nordman, M. & Pollock, M. (1998). Effects of 6 months of high- or low-volume resistance training on muscular strength and endurance. *Medicine and Science in Sports and Exercise*, *30* (suppl), S165.
	Fincher, G. E. (2000). The effect of high intensity resistance training on peak upper and lower body power among collegiate football players. *Medicine and Science in Sports and Exercise*, *32*

(suppl), S152.

Hass, C. J., Garzarella, L., De Hoyos, D. & Pollock, M. L. (2000). Single versus multiple sets in long-term recreational weightlifters. *Medicine and Science in Sports and Exercise, 3,* 235-242.

Jacobson, B. H. (1986). A comparison of two progressive weight training techniques on knee extensor strength. *Athletic Training, 21,* 315-318, 390.

Kosmahl, E. M., Mackarey, P. J. & Buntz, S. E. (1989). Nautilus training system versus traditional weight training system. *Journal of Orthopaedic and Sports Physical Therapy, 11,* 253-258.

Larshus, J. L., Hoeger, W. W. K. & Moore, J. R. (1997). Effects of multiple exercise training on the development of tricep strength. *Research Quarterly for Exercise and Sport,* Mar (suppl), A33-4.

Leighton, J. R., Holmes, D., Benson, J., Woolen, B. & Schmerer, R. (1967). A study of the effectiveness of ten different methods of progressive resistance exercise on the development of strength, flexibility, girth and bodyweight. *Journal of the Association of Physical and Mental Rehabilitation, 21,* 78-81.

Messier, S. P. & Dill, M. E. (1985). Alterations in strength and maximal oxygen uptake consequent to Nautilus circuit weight training. *Research Quarterly for Exercise and Sport, 56,* 345-351.

Pollock, M. L., Abe, T., De Hoyos, D. V., Garzarella, L., Hass, C. J. & Werber, G. (1998). Muscular hypertrophy responses to 6 months of high- or low-volume resistance training. *Medicine and Science in Sports and Exercise, 30* (suppl),

S116.

Reid, C. M., Yeater, R. A. & Ullrich, I. H. (1987). Weight training and strength, cardiorespiratory functioning and body composition. *British Journal of Sports Medicine*, *21*, 40-44.

Sanborn, K., Boros, R., Hruby, J., Schilling, B., O'Bryant, H. S., Johnson, R. L., Hoke, T., Stone, M. E. & Stone, M. H. (2000). Short-term performance effects of weight training with multiple sets not to failure vs. a single set to failure in women. *The Journal of Strength and Conditioning Research*, *14*, 328-331.

Silvester, L. J., Stiggins, C., McGown, C. & Bryce, G. R. (1982). The effect of variable resistance and free-weight training programs on strength and vertical jump. *National Strength and Conditioning Association Journal*, *3*, 30-33.

Starkey, D. B., Pollock M. L., Ishida, Y., Welsch, M. A., Brechue, W. F., Graves, J. E. & Feigenbaum, M. S. (1996). Effect of resistance training volume on strength and muscle thickness. *Medicine and Science in Sports and Exercise*, *28*, 1311-1320.

Stowers, T., McMillan, J., Scala, D., Davis, V., Wilson, D. & Stone, M. (1983). The short-term effects of three different strength-power training methods. *National Strength and Conditioning Association Journal*, *5*, 24-27.

Terbizan, D. J. & Bartels, R. I. (1985). The effect of set-repetition combinations on strength gain in females age 18-35. *Medicine and Science in Sports and Exercise*, *17* (suppl), S267.

Vincent, K., De Hoyos, D., Garzarella, L., Hass, C., Nordman, M. & Pollock, M. (1998). Relationship between indices of knee extension strength before and after training. *Medicine and Science in*

	Sports and Exercise, 30 (suppl), S163.
	Welsch, M. A., Brechue, W. F., Pollock, M. L., Starkey, D. B. & Graves, J. B. (1994). Effect of reduced training volume on bilateral isometric knee/extension torque. *Medicine and Science in Sports and Exercise, 26* (suppl), S189.
1,2, and 3	Berger, R. A. (1972). Effect of varied sets of static training on dynamic strength. *American Corrective Therapy Journal, 26* (2), 52-54.
	Rowles, M. P., Barnard, K. L., Adams, K. J., et al. (2000). Single vs. multiple set strength training in male phase II cardiac patients. *Medicine and Science in Sports and Exercise, 32* (suppl), S91.
	Stone, W. J. & Coulter, S. P. (1994). Strength/endurance effects from three resistance training protocols with women. *The Journal of Strength and Conditioning Research, 8,* 231-234.
	Westcott, W. L., Greenberger, K. & Milius, D. (1989). Strength training research: sets and repetitions. *Scholastic Coach, 58,* 98-100.
1,2, and 4	Ostrowski, K. J., Wilson, G. J., Weatherby, R., Murphy, P. W. & Lyttle, A. D. (1997). The effect of weight training volume on hormonal output and muscular size and function. *The Journal of Strength and Conditioning Research, 11,* 148-154.
2 and 3	Stadler, L. V., Stubbs, N. B. & Vukovich, M. D. (1997). A comparison of a 2-day and 3-day per week resistance training program on strength gains in older adults. *Medicine and Science in Sports and Exercise, 29* (suppl), S254.
2, 3 and 4	Luecke, T., Wendeln, H., Campos, G. R., Hagerman, F. C., Hikida, R. S. & Staron, R. S. (1998). The effects of three different resistance

	training programs on cardiorespiratory function. *Medicine and Science in Sports and Exercise, 30* (suppl), S198.
3 and 6	Berger, R. A. (1963). Comparative effects of three weight training programs. *The Research Quarterly, 34*, 396-398.
	Chestnut, J. L. & Docherty, D. (1999). The effects of 4 and 10 repetition maximum weight-training protocols on neuromuscular adaptations in untrained men. *The Journal of Strength and Conditioning Research, 13*, 353-359.
3, 4, and 5	Withers, R. T. (1970). Effect of varied weight-training loads on the strength of university freshmen. *The Research Quarterly, 41*, 110-114.
3, 5, and 7	Schmidtbleicher, D. & Buehrle, M. (1987). Neuronal adaptation and increase of cross-sectional area studying different strength training methods. In B. Jonsson (Ed.), *Biomechanics X-B* (pp. 615-620). Champaign, IL: Human Kinetics.
3, 6, and 8	Wenzel, R. R. & Perfetto, E. M. (1992). The effect of speed versus non-speed training in power development. *Journal of Applied Sports Science Research, 6*, 82-87.
5-6 and 8-9	Hisaeda, H., Miyagawa, K., Kuno, S., Fukunaga, T. & Muraoka, I. (1996). Influence of two different modes of resistance training in female subjects. *Ergonomics, 39*, 842-852.
5 and 10	Dudley, G. A., Tesch, P. A., Miller, M. A. & Buchanan, M. D. (1991). Importance of eccentric actions in performance adaptations to resistance training. *Aviation, Space, and Environmental Medicine, 62*, 543-550.

5 and 15	Ciriello, V. M., Holden, W. L. & Evans, W. J. (1982). The effects of two isokinetic training regimens on muscle strength and fiber composition. In H. G. Knuttgen, J. A. Vogel & J. Poortmans (Eds.), *Biochemistry of exercise* (pp. 787-793). Champaign, IL: Human Kinetics.

In an overview entitled *Evidence-based resistance training recommendations for muscular hypertrophy* the authors James Fisher, James Steele and Dave Smith state that "single set training appears to provide similar hypertrophic gains to multiple set training" and emphasize the importance of training to momentary muscular failure. They conclude that "evidence supports that persons should train to the highest intensity of effort, thus recruiting as many motor units and muscle fibers as possible, self-selecting a load and repetition range, and performing single sets for each exercise" [23].

Considering the lack of evidence supporting multiple-set training, why is three-set training so widespread?

6　The Holy Trinity: All good things come in threes

There is a distinct cultural bias concerning the number three. Three is and has been a very special number throughout the history of mankind. There are three dimensions that we can perceive. According to Pythagoras three is the noblest of all digits and consists of the sum of all the numbers below it, symbolizing the beginning, the middle, and the end. The Latin phrase *omne trium perfectum*, meaning "everything that comes in threes is perfect", has found its way into most languages. Phrases like "three time's a charm", "third time's a charm" or "all good things come in threes" are often used in English and so is "aller guten Dinge sind drei" in German, "jamais deux sans trios" in French, "todo lo bueno viene trios'" in Spanish and so on. The Chinese consider three to be the perfect number.

In most religions three is the most important number.

In Christianity there is the Holy Trinity: the Father, the Son, and the Holy Spirit. God is almighty because of omniscience, omnipresence, and omnipotence. Life consists of three stages: life, death, and rebirth.

The number three is mentioned more than 500 times in the Bible whereas every other number is mentioned fewer than ten times.

Some well-known examples of the number three in the bible are: Jesus met three great temptations in the desert. He said to Peter: "This very night, before the rooster crows, you will disown me three times." Jesus fell three times when carrying his cross. Three days after being crucified Jesus rose from the dead. Also, there are three theological virtues (Faith, Hope, and Charity) and three attributes of the Christ (I am the way, the truth, and the life).

The number three represents the three aspects of human life: material, rational and spiritual.

Life itself consists of birth, life, and death.

There are three primary colors, of which all other colors can be produced.

Our planet's surface consists of one third land and two thirds water.

There are three dimensions that we can perceive (height, width, and depth) and three states of matter (gas, solid, liquid).

Time consists of the past, the present, and the future.

The separation of powers calls for three branches: legislative, executive, and judiciary.

The three inalienable rights voiced in the U.S. Declaration of Independence are life, liberty, and the pursuit of happiness. The motto of the French revolution was: *Liberté, Egalité,* and *Fraternité.* The German national anthem is about *Einigkeit, und Recht, und Freiheit* (unity, justice, and liberty). Julius Caesar wrote to the Roman Senate: *"veni, vidi, vici"* ("I came, saw, and won") and Shakespeare had his literary Julius Caesar address his audience with "friends, Romans, countrymen."

According to Freud, the human personality as a whole consists of id, ego, and super-ego.

A good story consists of a beginning, a middle part, and an end.

Most abbreviations consist of three letters, for example: CNN, ABC, BBC, CBC, NHK, WWW, USA, JFK, FBI, CIA, NSA, CEO, CFO, OMG, LOL, USD, GPD, EUR, JPY, JPG, MP3, CPU, ROM, RAM, DOS, and many others. The alphabet, consisting of 26 letters, is called "the ABC".

You arrive early, late, or on time.

In an auction the auctioneer says: "going once, going twice, sold" or "going, going, gone".

There are three basic meals a day: breakfast, lunch, and dinner (often consisting of appetizer, main course, and dessert). Food consists of three macronutrients: protein, carbohydrates, and fat.

Even in jokes, there usually is a trichotomy: "An Englishmen, an Irishman, and a Scotsman...".

"There once was a farmer who had three sons...". Santa Claus says "ho, ho, ho", Superman "up, up, and away".

The three wise monkeys, three little pigs, the three bears, three wishes for Cinderella, three witches in Shakespeare's Macbeth ("Thrice the brindled cat hath mewed"), three measurements (hip, waist, and chest), the three musketeers, three phases of the moon.

Grammar consists of three persons, three numbers, three genders, and three degrees of comparison ("good – better – best").

Also, three is the most important number in philosophy. Aristotele regarded the triad as the number of the complete whole. Compte believed that there are three phases of development that the human mind goes through. Kant saw three principles of homogeneity. Hegel's dialectic consists of thesis, antithesis, and synthesis.

You could spend your money for wine, women, and song. Or you could invest in real estate instead, but if you do, you will be advised that there are three things that matter: location, location, and location. It is a rule of thumb in economics that there are usually three major competitors in any free market. There are three work shifts: morning shift, late shift, and night shift.

Two people moving a piece of furniture will lift it "on the count of three".

I could go on, and on, and on...

I will give you three guesses what my point is: The number three has an outstanding cultural significance, a positive bias that no other number can match.

And this is the truth, the whole truth and nothing but the truth.

The number three in sports

This significance of the number three is also prevalent in sports.

- The Olympic motto is *citius*, *altius*, and *fortius*.

- In baseball there are three bases, three strikes before a batter is out and three outs for each team in each inning.

- In basketball there is the "three-second rule", and a successful shot from a certain distance is worth three points.

- In boxing each round takes three minutes, and the ring is surrounded by three ropes. In most organizations a fight is judged by three judges.

- There are three exercises in powerlifting: the deadlift, the bench press, and the squat.

- In weightlifting competitions each competitors has three attempts and there are three judges.

- To win in wrestling one has to put the opponent on his shoulders for a count of three.

- In all kinds of sport winning a match is celebrated by three cheers, each consisting of three shouts like "hip, hip, hooray". In athletics the command is threefold: "on your mark, get set, go". The first three finishers receive a medal (bronze, silver, and gold).

- In football (soccer), the world's most popular sport, there is a win, a loss, or a draw. The team receives three points for a win and three players can be replaced in a match. Also, there are three tactical areas (defense, midfield and offence) and three referees on the pitch (a head referee and two linesmen).

- In sports a hat-trick consists of a series of three goals. The greatest success a team can possibly achieve is the "triple", consisting of winning the national league, the national cup, and the champions' league.

Three-set training

Considering this widespread cultural bias of the number three, also prevalent in sports, it is hardly surprising that, since there were no evidence-based training guidelines, three-set training became the norm. Arnold Schwarzenegger writes in his autobiography that when he started training as a teenager there wasn't really any information available on how to train for muscle growth but his mentors who had been training since the 1950s recommended doing multiple sets of each exercise [24]. Later Schwarzenegger himself became the role-model for thousands, if not millions of trainees who copied his multiple-set training hoping to be as successful with it as he was.

When the Berger study was published in 1962 most people found it plausible that multiple sets were better than "just" one set and three sets of each exercise were considered to be the perfect number of sets for optimum results, even though there was no supporting evidence from a scientific point of view.

Despite this lack of scientific information on training, there is another deficiency: the absence of logic behind the concept of "the more, the better" and "third time's a charm":

If two sets are said to be better than one set and three sets better than two sets, why are then three sets better than four? Does the "the more, the better" concept not imply that four sets are even better than three? Some coaches and scholars obviously thought so.

In a very popular bestselling book on designing resistance training programs from 1987 the authors state that "the number of sets used in a workout is directly related to training results" [25]. Here again, the concept of "the more, the better" occurs. This raises another question: If "the number of sets in a workout is directly related to training results" why should three sets then be the ideal number of sets? According to this logic, more sets would be even better. Six sets would produce better results than three.

Obviously, proponents of three-set training do not apply their own logic. They do not offer any explanation why three sets are better than two and much better than one set, yet more than three sets are *not* better. If the number of sets is "directly related to training results", why should we stop after doing three sets and not do thirty-three sets or even three-hundred-thirty-three?

If the volume of exercise was essential to make muscles grow, marathon runners would definitely be more muscular than sprinters.

The (unfounded) logic of "more sets are better" apparently only applies to number of sets between zero and three with three being the optimum (*omne trium perfectum*). Applying the same logic to other kinds of aspects of human physiology would translate into the following recommendations:

1. If taking 200mg of a medicine a day will help you to get well within two weeks, then taking 400mg a day will make you well within one week. And taking 600 mg a day will make sure you will be fine in a few days (in 3.5 days to be precise).

2. One hour a day in the Mediterranean midday sun will get you a tan, two hours a day will make you twice as tanned and three hours will get you an optimum tan.

3. Taking one birth control pill every day will make it impossible to become pregnant. Taking two birth control pills a day will make it more impossible to become pregnant. Taking three birth control pills will make it most impossible to become pregnant.

4. If you get a vaccination against a certain disease, you will be immune. After getting another vaccination two or three minutes later, you will be even more immune and three vaccinations will make you most immune against that disease.

The same absurdity of that logic is the point in the old joke about the man whose mother-in-law died. He calls the local undertaker and discusses the funeral with him. The undertaker tells him: "There are three options: a simple funeral, burial at sea, and cremation." The man thinks for a moment and then he says: "Okay, do all three, take no chances."

There is a reason why there is neither a comparative nor superlative of words like pregnant, immune, or dead. They describe an either/or condition. Our body either adapts to a certain stimulus or does not. There is no condition in between. It is like flipping a light switch. If you put your finger on it, you must produce enough pressure for the switch to move. If you do, the light is switched on and there is no need to do it a second or third time. If you don't, the light switch will not move and the light remains unlit.

If the training stimulus is adequate and surpasses the necessary threshold, the corresponding adaptation is induced. This is exactly what High Intensity Training does.

7   The paradigm shift that never happened

High Intensity Training has been around since the 1970s. Several studies have shown its outstanding efficiency and thousands of people world-wide have made great progress with this kind of training method. High Intensity Training is very popular in medical circles. Some of the best athletes and bodybuilders in the world owe their success to High Intensity Training and evidence-based training guidelines now recommend intense single-set training. Yet three-set training is still the norm. The paradigm shift from high volume training to High Intensity Training that some have predicted based on the proven efficiency of HIT, has not yet taken place and is not likely to do so any time soon for several reasons:

The Semmelweis-reflex

Newly discovered insights that contradict established norms and paradigms are usually rejected.

Three-set training became the norm in the 1960s and still is. Millions of people world-wide follow the recommendation to train with multiple sets of each exercise, preferably three. All the information available now that shows that it is intensity rather than volume that makes muscles grow is often ignored or even rejected.

Rejecting new information that contradicts established norms is called the Semmelweis-reflex. Ignaz Semmelweis was a medical doctor working in a hospital in Vienna, Austria, during the 19th century. In 1847 Dr. Semmelweis discovered that the maternal mortality rate due to puerperal fever could be decreased dramatically if doctors washed their hands with chlorinated lime solutions after autopsy work before treating their patients. When Semmelweis made doctors in his hospital also sterilize the medical instruments with the same chlorinated solution the mortality rate (formerly 7% to 16% before Semmelweis' discovery) dropped to 1% [26]. Semmelweis expected his recommendations would be followed by his colleagues all over the country, thereby saving thousands of lives. Instead, Semmelweis' suggestions were strongly rejected by the scientific community at that time because they contradicted the then prevailing belief that infections were caused by either a "disharmony of body fluids" like "phlegm" or "black bile", or by "miasma" (a kind of "bad air"), as every doctor had been taught at university during that time. Instead of being invited to teach doctors hygiene, Semmelweis was openly criticized, even ridiculed. He later lost his job and was finally put in an insane asylum where he died at age 47.

There are other similar extreme examples from the past and more in the present. Nicolaus Copernicus found out that the earth revolved around the Sun and not vice versa. He published his heliocentric model in 1543. One hundred years later school children and university students were still taught that the earth was the centre of the universe and the sun revolved around the earth. Galileo Galilei was even taken to court and forced to abrogate his statement that the earth was not the centre of the universe. And that was more than half a century after Copernicus' discovery!

When Alfred Wegener presented his theory of continental drift at the annual meeting of the Geological Association in Frankfurt, Germany in January 1912, several of the geologists in attendance burst out laughing. There was a consensus that his theory was "ridiculous". Wegener knew that it would not be easy to convince the scientific community, but was not quite prepared for the vehemence of the rejection, which was belligerent and even hateful. However, Wegener was convinced that his theory of continental drift was accurate. He presented supporting evidence and arguments and was sure that his theory would gain acceptance within the next ten years. But the theory of continental drift was dismissed by the scientific community. Even three decades later, the *American Journal of Science* published an article in which one of the leading paleontologists vehemently attacked Wegener and tried to prove that "most of the arguments supporting the drift hypothesis are shown to be based on erroneous conceptions" [27]. English broadcaster and naturalist David Attenborough once said in a newspaper interview that when he was a university student in the late 1940s he asked one of the lecturers why he never mentioned continental drift and was told that Wegener's concept was obviously "moonshine".

In the late 1960s after further research on the theory of plate tectonics, the theory of continental drift finally became generally accepted as valid. That was more than 30 years after Alfred Wegener's death.

Tradition

Usually, most professors, lecturers, P.E. teachers, successful athletes, and coaches teach what they have been taught, which is that multiple sets are better than "just" one set, that three sets are best, that the more experienced you become the more often you must train and that more volume is required to improve further.

One prominent example: The authors of the aforementioned best-selling book from 1987 on designing resistance training programs who wrote that results were "directly related to exercise volume", published an updated fourth edition of their book in 2014 in which they paraphrased their statement from 1987 only slightly: "A relationship exists between higher training volumes and training outcomes, such as muscle hypertrophy, decreased body fat, increased fat-free mass, and even motor performance" [28]. They further claim that one set of an exercise was not enough to make any progress: "...studies support the contention that training volume greater than one set is needed for improvement and progression in physical development and performance, especially after the initial training period starting from the untrained state" [29].

On a side-note: One of the studies the authors list as a reference to support their opinion is the Berger study from 1962!

However, a study published in 2014 clearly showed that trained individuals who performed one set to muscular failure considerably improved both strength and body composition [30]. Not only did they build muscle but they also lost a significant amount of body fat.

The statement that one intense training set is not sufficient is not only unsubstantiated, it is also illogical. If one set does *not* generate improvement, which means it does nothing in terms of "improvement and progression in physical development and performance", how then can several sets of nothing lead to better results? If one set is useless, how many times do you have to repeat this kind of useless effort for maximal improvement? Three times, presumably.

More importantly, the quotation above shows that in the new edition (2014) of a very influential book on designing resistance training programs the authors still claim that "progression in physical development and performance" requires multiple-set training. This again will influence many scholars, P.E. teachers, and coaches who will then continue to recommend multiple-set training now and in the future.

The self-fulfilling tautology

The popularity of multiple-set training, especially three-set training, creates a kind of self-fulfilling tautology. The argument for three-set training could look like this:

a) *Everybody does three sets because this is the best way to train.*

b) *Since everybody does three sets, this must indeed be the best way to train.*

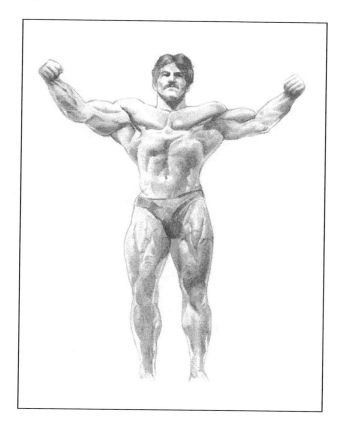

Figure 11: Mike Mentzer

This tautology is used very often in bodybuilding magazines and has even found its way into the scientific discourse. In the 1990s Mike Mentzer, a former Mr. Universe who won his title by applying Arthur Jones' concept of High Intensity Training to his training, wrote an article in a bodybuilding magazine in which he explained that one set of each exercise is enough to make muscles grow, provided that this set is taken to muscular failure. When the article appeared in print, the publisher included several photos of very big bodybuilders on the same pages of the article, along with a reference to their high-volume training programs under the headline "Is everyone really wrong?" [31]. The reference implies that the high-volume approach must be the best way to train because "everybody" uses it. This gives the readers of the magazine the impression that "every" successful professional bodybuilder does a lot of volume, which is not the case at all.

This argument was even brought up in the scientific discourse on single-set vs. multiple-set training. In 1997 an article was published in which the authors state that single-set training may be suitable for beginners whereas advanced trainees would improve more doing multiple sets [32]. The authors conclude that multiple-set training would not have become the prevalent training method among bodybuilders if single-set training produced comparable gains of muscle mass.

This argument is questionable for several reasons. First of all, we know that three-set training became the norm in bodybuilding just because there was no scientific research available that the bodybuilders could have relied on. So they chose a number that they were comfortable with. Not surprisingly, they chose the number that has the most positive cultural connotation: the number three.

Claiming that a certain way of doing something was best because most people believe it to be so; is not exactly a convincing argument.

Not too long ago, most people believed that the sun revolved around the earth, which was presumed to be flat, by the way. This is like saying that the best day for a car wash is Saturday because that is when most people clean their car.

Imagine a scientific discourse about our solar system in which someone argues that the earth could not revolve around the Sun because so many people for so long were convinced of the opposite.

There are people who believe that they can cause rainfall by dancing. If the number of people who believe this exceeds one or two million should this make us question the proven laws of meteorology?

The authors of the article about single-set training conceded that doing one set per exercise was okay for beginners but claimed that advanced athletes needed multiple-set training to make progress. Ironically, the article was written only a few years after competitive bodybuilding had been dominated for more than half a decade by British bodybuilder Dorian Yates and his High Intensity Training, a fact that was completely ignored by the authors.

Neomania

We all have a tendency to always look for something new. When we read that a new improved version of the car we are driving or the computer we are using is now available, we may want to have it. It is not unusual for people to buy a new cell phone every two years. Very often, a new device is better than the old one. Sometimes it only looks more attractive.

Fashion trends come and go. Some people like to enjoy a similar variety in sports and physical activity. And there is a wide range of sports activities to choose from. The list goes from A as in Aerobics to Z as in Zumba and everything in between. And there is nothing wrong with that. Variety is the proverbial spice of life. But again, we must be careful not to mix the terms playing, practicing, being active, and doing sports with *training* because training is something completely different. It is a very specific process that must fulfill certain criteria in order to be successful.

Some people might try HIT for a while because they consider it "hot" and "new" and later will move on to something even "hotter" and "newer". For sure there will soon be some new, innovative, and revolutionary training method with a fitting acronym, maybe something like "Basic Universal Light Load Super Hyper Innovative Training". This will lead to the marketing of training equipment, food supplements, several clothing collections, computer programs and apps one "must have" to participate in that brand new hot training program.

But High Intensity Training is not just a passing trend. It is neither "hot" nor "new". It has been around since the 1970s and its roots reach back more than two thousand years. Besides, High Intensity Training is not just another kind of training. It is the practical application of training science. HIT makes sure that the desired adaptations of the human body take place by triggering them adequately and by allowing enough rest and recuperation to let the body supercompensate.

Reversing the burden of proof

Usually, if someone wants you to do *more*, he or she has to bring up convincing arguments. If your boss wants you to work more, if your doctor wants you to take more medicine, if your wife wants you to spend more time with your mother-in-law, if your kids want more pocket-money, they all better have some good arguments to convince you. Would you work three times as many hours each week for the same salary? Well, most people would not. But when it comes to training, things are turned upside down. Although many studies have shown that increasing the number of sets in a workout will *not* produce significantly better results (see the list of studies on pages 61-68), many people work out three times as much as actually necessary, risking overtraining and health problems, not questioning what they are doing because "everybody" works out like that. This has created a paradox. Those who decide to perform one sufficiently intense set per exercise – the kind of training that is based on the physiological process of how the human body adapts to stimuli – are expected to justify their decision. Those who decide to work out three times as much as necessary do not need to prove their point since this is common practice.

Misinformation

A lot of misinformation about HIT is still in circulation. There are four points that need to be addressed in this context:

"HIT is dangerous because you have to use very heavy weights"

The opposite is true. HIT is not about lifting very heavy weights, it is about stimulating the muscles as much as possible. In order to do so, each repetition must be performed very slowly and in perfect form. The concentric phase of a repetition (i.e. lifting the weight upwards) has to take at least two seconds. At the fully contracted position the weight is held statically for a second and then lowered very slowly which takes another three to four seconds. In sum repetitions take at least seven seconds. This completely avoids momentum and makes sure that the target muscles are doing the work.

The misinformation about High Intensity Training being dangerous goes back to a time when the term "intensity" had not yet been defined properly for resistance training. In aerobic training, intensity is usually measured by counting heartbeats per minute and relating that number to the individual's maximum heart rate. For example, someone whose maximum heart rate is 200 beats per minute exercises at an intensity level of 80% when his heart rate is 160 beats per minute and exercises at an intensity level of 90% when his heart beats 180 times per minute.

In the past, a similar approach was used for resistance training. Intensity was measured by how close the *weights* lifted were to the one-repetition maximum, i.e. the amount of weight can be lifted only once, like in weightlifting. The heavier the weights, the higher the intensity. A definition like this is rather inappropriate, as the following example shows. If someone bench pressed 100 pounds for ten repetitions, by that definition the intensity would be considered higher than if the same person benched 99 pounds twenty times, just because the weight was heavier. This approach does not consider *intensity of effort*.

It cannot be said often enough: High Intensity Training is not about lifting very heavy weights, it is about slowly and safely lifting moderate resistances to momentary muscular failure.

"Doing only one set is okay for beginners but advanced trainees need to do substantially increase training volume"

If this statement was true, the most advanced athletes in the world, like Olympic champions, would need to do hundreds or even thousands of sets. Training must indeed be progressive, but increasing the number of sets is not the answer.

It is not unusual to gain several percent of strength each month, especially for beginners. Adding only one set per exercise every five weeks (which is not much in terms of progression) would add up to having to do more than 100 sets per exercise ten years later. Someone starting at fifteen and reaching his peak at around 35 years would then have to do *over two hundred sets* – of each exercise!

Proponents of multiple-set training often argue that doing multiple sets per exercise were the reason for the great success of Arnold Schwarzenegger, the most successful bodybuilder of all times. However, one look at his famous training methods shows that this is not the case. In fact, Schwarzenegger did *not* increase his training volume as he progressed.

We know from his autobiography that he did up to ten sets per exercise as a beginner [24] and between four to six sets when he trained for the Mr. Universe and Mr. Olympia contests. If it is necessary to increase the number of sets as one progresses, how many more sets would have been necessary for Schwarzenegger to become as successful as he has?

Those people who claim that Arnold Schwarzenegger became the most successful bodybuilder in history "because he trained up to five hours a day" should try to become even better than he was by training not five, but six or seven hours a day.

What some people misunderstand when they argue that advanced trainees need to do "more" is that training indeed has to be progressive but increasing training volume is only *one* way to make training progressive. And it is not the best one. You will soon reach an amount of training volume that is impossible to do and too much to recover from.

A more sensible approach is to progressively increase the resistance. This is what Milo did more than two thousand years ago. Milo could have carried a calf twice or three times a day. Instead he took advantage of the fact that the calf he carried every day gained weight daily. Accordingly, the resistance he dealt with increased. However, once you can lift 50 pounds ten times then you could of course do more sets. A better way to make your training progressive is to either try to do eleven repetitions or to increase the resistance by a few per cent and try to still do ten repetitions.

This is exactly what Schwarzenegger did. While it is true that Arnold Schwarzenegger usually did more than one set of an exercise, he always pointed out: "Intensity was the key to my bodybuilding success, regardless of what muscle group I was training" [33].

As explained before, high intensity of effort triggers muscle growth and Arnold Schwarzenegger was well aware of that as he pointed out: "One of the best-kept secrets about training is that maximum effort is required to make maximum gains. (...) Each set should be taken to muscular failure and beyond ..." [34].

"You cannot train HIT unless you have access to special training equipment"

Training equipment like special training "machines" help to keep proper form while lifting. The term "machine" is to some extend misleading in this context because a machine is usually associated with something that moves you, like a car for example. In this case the trainee moves the "machine". Another advantage of training with a "machine" is that one does not have to worry about getting a barbell off one's chest after reaching the point of momentary muscular failure. However, this does not mean that those machines are necessary for High Intensity Training. The inventor of those machines,

Arthur Jones, always pointed out that the principles underlying High Intensity Training are universal and of course do also apply to training with traditional training equipment like barbells, dumbbells, dipping bars and so forth. Arthur Jones himself used traditional equipment in the beginning:

"I built my greatest size and strength with nothing more than a barbell, a squat rack, a chinning bar, and a pair of parallel dip bars – all of which equipment is available to almost anybody for a few dollars, and none of which pieces of equipment are manufactured by my company." [35]

The principles of High Intensity Training are universal and can even be applied to body weight exercises like push-ups or chin ups, not requiring any equipment at all.

"Training to muscular failure should be avoided."

Failure is not a four letter word. Some people do not like the idea of training to muscular failure before they have even tried to do so. This attitude is just as understandable as it is widespread. The term "training to the point of momentary muscular failure" contains a word that evokes the most negative associations one can think of. Which word could possibly sound worse than the word "failure"? In almost every other context the word describes something negative, meaning that a certain endeavor was *not* successful, that an aim could *not* be reached. In the context of training the opposite is true. Training to the point of momentary muscular failure means that the trainee was successful in reaching his or her best possible performance. If you fail in doing another repetition, you have succeeded in giving the very best you are capable of, making sure you have created a powerful stimulus that passes the necessary threshold and thus triggers the desired adaptations in your body.

The final repetitions are crucial. Not doing them for fear of "failure" is just as paradox as taking only 50 milligrams of a vaccine that only works at a dose of 150 milligrams. It does not mean to just miss out on "some" of the desired effects, it means not getting *any* result at all. Remember: the stimulus-reaction scheme describes an all-or-nothing situation. If the stimulus is insufficient, the desired reaction will not take place at all. On a cloudy November day, you can spend all day outside but will not get a tan since the stimulus is insufficient. But if the stimulus is sufficient by surpassing the necessary threshold, there will be the full reaction. And by training to momentary muscular failure, High Intensity Training certainly makes sure that the threshold is surpassed and the desired adaptations will take place.

As Albert Einstein once said "failure is success in progress". This is definitely true when it comes to training.

8   The essence of High Intensity Training

Training programs based on the principles of HIT can be seen as a practical application of the following guidelines:

- Focus on basic multi-joint exercises.
- Perform one set per exercise.
- Take each set to momentary muscular failure.
- Execute each repetition in perfect form and deliberately slowly, completely avoiding momentum.
- Choose a moderate weight and aim for reaching muscular failure within a time under tension of about 60 to 120 seconds (six to twelve slow repetitions).
- Make your training progressive by trying to increase the number of repetitions with the same resistance.
- Increase resistance when you can do more than twelve slow repetitions (or when time under tension exceeds 120 seconds).
- Train once, twice or three times a week depending on whether or not you use a split routine.
- Take enough rest enough between workouts to let the body recover and adapt to the training stimulus by over-compensating.
- Take additional days off if you feel inadequately recovered.
- Take a full week off if you feel overtrained.
- Consume a well-balanced diet containing between 1.5 to 2 grams of protein per kilogram of bodyweight.

- Do not take drugs.

Safety

HIT is very safe. It is important that every repetition of every exercise is completed very slowly and in perfect style, completely avoiding momentum. Another reason why HIT is safe is that special attention is paid to the first repetition of each set. Doing so avoids the dangerous, yet widespread habit of starting the first repetition of a set with a slight swing or kick to get the weight moving. Instead, the first repetition of a set begins several seconds before the weight actually starts moving. By gradually increasing isometric tension in the muscles needed for the execution of that particular lift, the weight does not start to move before the force of muscle contraction exceeds the weight of the resistance.

Let's look at the execution of a leg press, for example. First the trainee makes sure he is in the right position and everything is arranged the way it is supposed to be. Then he will contract his leg muscles until they produce enough force to get weight moving. The set has actually begun several seconds before someone could even see any motion.

This extremely careful approach to training has led some to the opinion that warming-up was not necessary at all. And under ideal conditions this may be true. If you train with state-of-the-art exercise machines using moderate poundage, perfect form and isometric tension before you actually start to move the weight, you may indeed not need to have a special "warm-up-procedure" before. If, however, you are training with free weights, especially heavy ones, this is a completely different matter. Nobody should get under a 300-pound squat bar without previously preparing the body for this task. But, generally speaking, a "warm-up marathon" is definitely not necessary. A sensible approach for a full-body workout, for example, may consist of one light, submaximal set of a pressing movement, a rowing movement, and a leg pressing exercise to elevate body temperature and to get the blood flowing in the trained muscles.

When training with free weights it is mandatory to have a spotter for some exercises. Whereas training to muscular failure on barbell curls is not problematic because you simply will not be able to lift the barbell once you have reached muscular failure, exercises like bench presses or squats should always be done with a spotter. Otherwise you might have difficulties in getting the barbell off the chest.

Choosing the right exercises

Compound multi-joint exercises should be preferred over "isolation" exercises. For example, leg presses or squats should be preferred over single-leg extensions or good mornings, if possible. This does not mean that isolation exercises are not beneficial, they simply involve much less muscle activation than the compound exercises leg presses and squats. The same applies to basic exercises like deadlifts, chin-ups, dips, rows, front presses and many others.

However, if for some reason one of these recommended exercises cannot be performed, there are still alternatives to chose from. If somebody cannot do squats, for example, because of a lower back problem, but can do leg presses, there is no need to worry about not being able to do squats. Some people cannot do chin-ups for reps because they are too heavy. It is a good idea to keep trying, of course, and to reduce body fat and increase strength by doing lat pull-downs. And if somebody – for whatever reason – cannot do bench presses, doing incline dumbbell presses instead is much better than leaving out pressing movements completely.

If recommended exercises are not possible, the principles of High Intensity Training can still be applied to any other exercise, whether it is an abdominal crunch, a biceps curl or any other kind of exercise.

Exercise order

Bigger muscles should always be trained before smaller muscles, especially if they are both involved in the same exercise. That may sound complicated but is rather simple in practice: Thighs, chest, shoulders and back should be trained before biceps, triceps or calves. The larger the muscle, the more energy is required to train it. If the smaller muscles are trained first, there might not be enough energy left to train one of the larger muscles, or several of the larger muscles.

Another aspect that has to be considered is muscle synergism, i.e. how different muscles work together during certain exercises. For example, it is not possible to do a pressing movement for the chest without involving the triceps muscles. A chinning or rowing movement for the back cannot be performed without contractions of the biceps. This means that biceps and triceps are also stimulated by doing certain compound multi-joint exercises for the upper body. Those who wish to include specific arm exercises in the training program like biceps curls or triceps extensions should do those after completing the exercises for chest, back, and shoulders.

Applying all three types of muscle contraction to each repetition

High Intensity Training takes advantage of the fact that there are three different types of muscle contraction that can be used to get the most out of each repetition. Muscle training is often just seen as "lifting weights" whereas there is, in fact, much more to it than just lifting. The term "muscle contraction" may imply that the muscle is always shortening while under tension. However, there are three different types of contraction: isometric, concentric, and eccentric contractions. Each repetition should consist of all three kinds of muscular tension. The trained muscle should be kept under tension during all three phases of the repetition while it shortens, lengthens, or remains the same length during execution.

As mentioned, each repetition should begin with as much *isometric* tension as necessary to get the weight moving. Then the weight is lifted (*concentric*) to the top position, held for a short moment (*isometric*) and then lowered very slowly (*eccentric*). Isometric strength is greater than concentric strength and eccentric strength is even greater than isometric strength. This means that we can still hold a weight that we cannot lift anymore and can still lower it once we can no longer hold it.

Let's say somebody is doing chin-ups. On the last repetition the person reaches concentric failure after pulling himself up about 80% of the way. Many people will then let themselves drop down into the bottom position and then walk away from the chinning bar. But that would mean wasting the most crucial part of the set. What should be done instead is:

    a) try to pull yourself up even further (thereby try to extend the concentric phase of the repetition)

    b) when that is not possible, hold yourself as long as you can in that position (isometric phase of the repetition)

    c) when that is no longer possible, resist the lowering for as long as possible (extending the eccentric phase of the repetition)

Training beyond concentric muscular failure

Executing the final repetition of each set in the way described fulfills the criteria of training beyond concentric momentary muscular failure. After reaching concentric failure the set is not terminated but followed by more isometric and then eccentric muscular tension.

There are some exercises in which such a procedure is rather difficult, for example the barbell bench press or the squat exercise. Finishing a set of those exercises when reaching muscular failure requires the help of a spotter who helps to rack the weight.

Those who wish to increase training intensity even more, for example very advanced trainees, have several options, like drop sets, pre-exhaustion or post-exhaustion.

Drop sets

Instead of terminating a set when reaching muscular failure, the resistance can be reduced immediately (usually ten to thirty percent, depending on the exercise and the individual) to perform a few additional repetitions and to extend muscular time under tension.

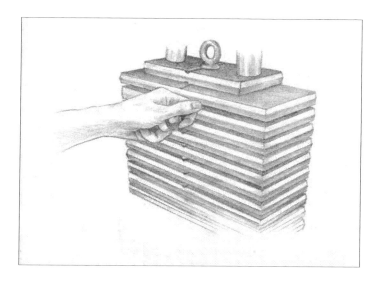

Figure 12: Drop set: reducing the resistance immediately after reaching muscular failure

In dumbbell training drop sets are also known as "working down the rack": The dumbbells are re-racked after reaching failure and a lighter pair of dumbbells is used to continue the set. Another expression for using drop sets in barbell exercises is "stripping", because the weight on the barbell is reduced by taking weight off each side. Extending time under tension by using drop sets is a good and safe way to train beyond muscular failure. For example, someone does an exercise using a resistance of 100 pounds. Reaching the point of momentary muscular failure means that the trainee's trained muscles have fatigued to the extent that the muscles are not capable of performing another repetition with 100 pounds. This does not mean that the muscles are so fatigued that they cannot move any weight at all anymore. In fact, the trainee may well be able to do a few additional repetitions with 80 or 75 pounds. And this is exactly what drop-set training takes advantage of.

Compound sets

A compound set consists of two exercises. Performed seamlessly after each other, they are considered one entity and can be counted as one set. Compound sets are used to compensate biomechanical limitations of training the target muscles by certain exercises. One characteristic example is the training of the chest muscles with a pressing movement like the bench press. Apart from the chest muscles several other muscles are working synergistically when executing this exercise, mainly lateral and frontal shoulders and triceps. Since the triceps are the weakest of the muscles involved in this exercise, they may fatigue before the chest muscles can be stimulated intensely enough. If this is the case, performing a compound set by combining a "flying" movement with a pressing movement for the chest offers a practical solution to overcome this problem. There are two different approaches to choose from: a pre-exhaustion compound set and a post-exhaustion compound set.

Pre-exhaustion

By performing a chest exercise with very little or no involvement of the triceps muscles, which is immediately followed by a chest pressing exercise, the pectoral muscles of the chest can be stimulated very intensely. When doing dumbbell flyes or pec-deck flyes before chest press, the muscles of the chest will already be exhausted to a large extent whereas the triceps will not. Therefore, the intensity of the pressing movement is not limited due to fatigued triceps muscles. Arthur Jones was aware of this problem when he designed his first exercise machines for high intensity training. He even created machines that allowed pec-deck flyes and chest presses in the same machine to keep the pause between the two exercises to the minimum. It used to be considered necessary to perform both exercises without any break between them. We know now that it takes the body about twenty seconds to restore around 50% of the ATP energy sources in the trained muscles and the completion of resynthesis of ATP in a fatigued muscle takes at least three minutes. This means that although changing from one exercise to the other should be as brief as possible to maximize the effect, it is not problematic if the process takes a few seconds. Anything less than 30 seconds would still be acceptable for the purpose of pre-exhausting the target muscle.

Post-exhaustion

Recently, a different kind of compound set has become very popular for High Intensity Training. Post-exhaustion is based on the same basic principle as pre-exhaustion but applies a reversed sequence. First the chest press exercise is performed, followed immediately by a "flying" movement. Applying post-exhaustion to back training, for example, would consist of performing a basic multi-joint exercise like the chin-up, rowing, or lat pull-downs immediately followed by a pullover exercise (either with a dumbbell, a barbell, or a machine) that requires little involvement of the biceps.

The advantage of post-exhaustion is that by reversing the order the basic multi-joint exercise is done when the target muscles are strongest. For example, after reaching failure on chin-ups (to which fatigue of the biceps may have contributed to a great extent) the back muscles are still kept under intense tension by doing pullovers to muscular failure. Post-exhaustion is particularly beneficial if somebody has difficulties in doing enough repetitions on exercises such as the chin-up. If somebody aims for ten repetitions but can only do six, post-exhausting the muscles by extending time under tension (e.g. by doing pullovers) makes perfect sense whereas pre-exhaustion would in this case be counterproductive since it would limit the number of chin-ups even further.

To split or not to split

HIT routines can either be full-body workouts or split programs. Each alternative offers certain advantages.

Advantages of full-body workouts

Full-body workouts train all the muscles of the body and let them all recuperate afterwards. This makes full-body workouts easy to schedule. If you cannot train on your usual training day, you simply train the next day. Instead of training, for example, on Mondays and Thursdays, you could just as well train on Tuesday and Friday or Wednesday and Saturday. Training your whole body in one session also takes advantage of muscle synergism. For example the biceps, too, are stressed when doing back exercises and the triceps are stimulated when training chest or shoulders. Only six to ten exercises are required to stimulate all parts of the body's musculature. Full-body workouts are great for beginners but are also an option for experienced trainees.

As discussed before, training is made progressive by increasing intensity, not volume. The time needed to complete the workout will not vary much between a beginner and an advanced trainee.

There is only one problem with full-body workouts. The physical work of one session might be so demanding and exhausting that it becomes difficult to keep intensity up throughout the whole workout. Training a large muscle group like the shoulders after already having trained the legs, back and chest can be very taxing, making it difficult to keep intensity up until the end of the workout. This is where split programs come into play.

Advantage of split programs

Training only particular muscle groups in each training session is less taxing on the whole system while allowing the trainee to apply high intensity throughout the workout. Unlike whole body programs that stress all the big muscles in the same workout, split programs usually target one or two of the big muscle groups in one session. Someone who has a hard time keeping intensity up until the end of a full-body workout may benefit enormously by splitting the routine into shorter sessions. By doing so each of the large muscle groups of the body like legs, back and chest can be trained at the beginning of the respective workout when energy levels are at their highest.

Regeneration is just as important as the workout itself

One thing that every trainee should be reminded of from time to time is that "muscles do not grow in the gym". This means that the workout itself merely serves as the trigger for muscle growth. To gain muscles the body must be given adequate rest afterwards. Once the muscles have completely recovered from the workout by not only compensating but even supercompensating the demands of the workout, the muscles will get stronger and bigger. Therefore it is imperative not to overtrain.

This inevitably begs the question "How much recovery time is necessary for supercompensation to take place?" Unfortunately there is no universal answer since recovery ability differs considerably between individuals. However, there is a good rule of thumb to go by. Each muscle should be trained either once or twice each week, which means that there should at least be two days of rest after a full-body workout and one day of rest after a workout that is part of a split routine.

When training the whole body in one session, training days could be Monday and Thursday, Monday and Friday, Tuesday and Friday, or

Tuesday and Saturday and so on, whereas a split routine could be performed on Monday, Wednesday and Friday or Tuesday, or Thursday, and Saturday, for example.

It is often claimed that experienced trainees need to train more often than beginners. This is not the case. Experienced trainees are able to train much more intensely using substantially more weight for the same number of repetitions than beginners. By doing so they put more stress on their bodies than beginners are capable of. Although an individual's recovery ability will indeed improve after years of training, recovery time is unlikely to decrease because of the much greater physical strain as a consequence of a much more demanding workout. For this reason training a muscle more often would be counterproductive.

Realistic expectations and comparisons

Just as with any other physiological process, there is also a limit to how much progress a person can make by training properly. Not everybody can grow to a height of seven feet or run as fast as an Olympic champion, even with the greatest training effort. Some people cannot get much of a suntan because of too little pigmentation in their skin. If they extend exposure time to the sun, they will burn their skin rather than get a tan.

The same genetic differences apply to muscle building. Those who have an abundance of muscle fibers and motor units will gain more muscle mass than those with a smaller number of muscle fibers and less favorable genetic conditions.

The only person you should compare yourself to is: yourself! Unless you have a monozygotic twin sibling comparing your own progress to someone else's does not make much sense. Instead, you should concentrate on improving yourself. And this is exactly what High Intensity Training implies.

In spite of what muscle magazines and food supplement companies tell us, no one – not even the more genetically gifted trainees – can become Mr. Universe or Miss Olympia overnight. A claim that someone built up thirty pounds of new muscle mass in a few months is unrealistic. Re-gaining muscle mass, however, is a different matter, as the Colorado Experiment and several other studies have shown. It is much easier and can be done much faster for the body to regain a physical condition it possessed earlier. This is good news for those who have been in shape before and are now trying to get back into that great shape they once had.

But High Intensity Training can also build new muscle mass very efficiently. For most people gaining a few pounds of new muscle mass every year while keeping body fat low must be considered a great success. Gains may well be greater during the first year when the body is still unaccustomed to the training stimulus but the more experienced a trainee becomes, the slower progress will be. Even then, High Intensity Training will result in steady progress that adds up to a success story over time. For example, just imagine someone gaining an average of three pounds of new muscles a year, more during the first years and less during the following years, this average gain of three pounds a year adding up to thirty pounds of new-built muscle within ten years will completely transform the physical condition.

HIT will make sure that the body receives adequate stimulation to continuously adapt and become bigger and stronger.

In the following chapter there are several suggestions for High Intensity Training programs to choose from and to adapt to your own individual needs.

9   Training programs

Taking all these facts together, one could easily come to the conclusion that designing training programs was a rather difficult task, but this is not the case. There is no need to make things more complicated than they are.

One reason why volume training is still so widespread is the (false) belief that to effectively train a certain muscle, it has to be "isolated". This means that the chosen exercises only train one particular muscle – and not any other muscles. To make things even more complicated, each muscle is said to be best developed by training it "from all angles", performing several different exercises for the same muscle. If those presumptions were true, it would literally take thousands of different exercises to effectively train all the muscles of the human body. There are more than 600 different skeletal muscles in the human body so we would at least need six-hundred different "isolation" exercises to address each muscle directly and even more exercises to train each muscle from several "angles".

Muscle synergism

Fortunately, this is completely unnecessary. It is possible to train all muscles with less than a dozen different exercises and the reason for this is muscle synergism. Whenever we execute a certain movement several muscles contract synergistically to make it happen. For example, several muscles of the arm contract together with the biceps when performing curls. Apart from those so-called prime movers, there are other muscles that contract to stabilize other parts of the body and keep joints in the necessary position for the execution of the lift. These muscles are called "fixators". A muscle that is trained as a prime mover during a certain exercise may serve as a fixator during another exercise and vice versa. This means that performing a few basic exercises will activate all the skeletal muscles of the body. Just think of the three exercises performed in powerlifting: deadlifts, bench presses, and squats. Which muscle of the body does not participate in one way or another to the execution of those lifts?

Sometimes, the phenomenon of muscle synergism becomes most apparent when muscle soreness occurs in muscles that were not at all intended to be the target muscles of the respective training session. Examples are sore triceps the day(s) following back training (one of the lesser-known functions of the triceps is to pull the arm back) and sore abdominals on day(s) following squats.

Each full-body workout should consist of:

- A pressing movement for the legs (leg presses, squats)
- A rowing or pulling movement for the back (lat pull-downs, pull-ups, chin-ups, rows)
- A pressing movement for the chest (bench presses, dips)
- An abdominal exercise (crunch, leg raises)

More exercises can be added like one or two additional leg exercises, a shoulder press, biceps curls, or triceps extensions. As a rule of thumb, the number of exercises should not exceed ten.

9.1 Sample full-body workout A

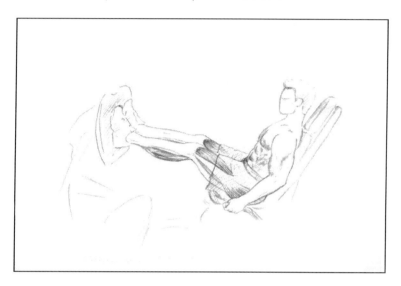

Figure 13: Leg press

Exercises

leg press
chest press
lat pull-down
leg curl
shoulder press
biceps curl
abdominal crunch

You can use the tables as a template to record the weight and the number of repetitions performed for each exercise and/or the time under tension until reaching muscle failure. Here is an example:

Date			
exercises	weight	reps	time under tension
leg press	198 lbs	12	82 sec
chest press	165 lbs	9	70 sec
lat pull-down	121 lbs	14	104 sec
leg curl	57 lbs	12	91 sec
shoulder press	40 lbs	11	82 sec
biceps curl	43 lbs	13	101 sec
abdominal crunch	--	15	118 sec

Date			
exercises	weight	reps	time under tension
leg press			
chest press			
lat pull-down			
leg curl			
shoulder press			
biceps curl			
abdominal crunch			

9.2   Sample full-body workout B

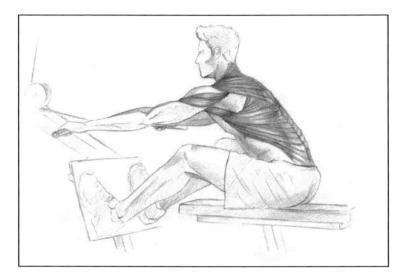

Figure 14: Back row

Exercises

squat
back row
incline chest press
leg extension
dips
leg curl
biceps curl
abdominal crunch

Date			
exercises	weight	reps	time under tension
squat			
back row			
incline chest press			
leg extension			
dips			
leg curl			
biceps curl			
abdominal crunch			

9.3   Sample full-body workout C

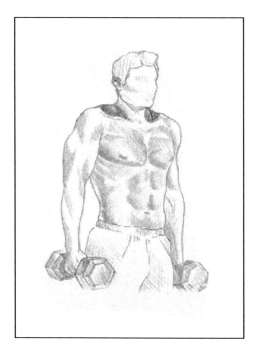

Figure 15: Shrug

Exercises

leg press
leg curl
dips
chin-up
dumbbell curl
shoulder press
shrug
leg raise

Date			
exercises	weight	reps	time under tension
leg press			
leg curl			
dips			
chin-up			
dumbbell curl			
shoulder press			
shrug			
leg raise			

9.4 Sample full body workout with pre-exhaustion A

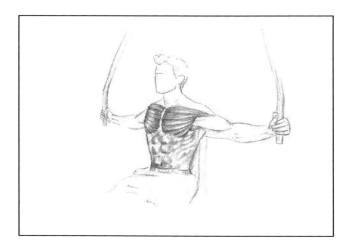

Figure 16: Pec-deck fly

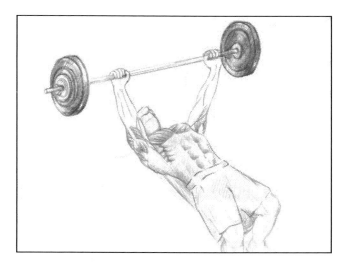

Figure 17: Incline bench press

Exercises

compound set of pec-deck fly and incline bench press
compound set of leg extension and leg press
compound set of cable pullover and lat pull-down
compound set of leg curl and calf raise

The total number of exercises should not exceed ten. If, for example, four compound sets are performed, additional sets should be limited to no more than two.

Date			
exercises	weight	reps	time under tension
ped-deck fly			
incline bench press			
leg extension			
leg press			
cable pullover			
lat pull-down			
leg curl			
calf raise			

9.5 Sample full body workout with pre-exhaustion B

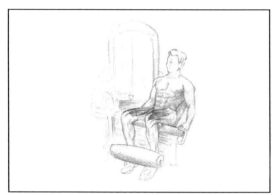

Figure 18: Leg extension

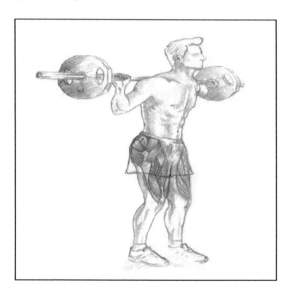

Figure 19: Squat

Exercises

compound set of leg extension and squat
compound set of dumbbell pullover and chin-up
compound set of dumbbell fly and bench press
biceps curl
lying leg curl
calf raise
abdominal crunch

Date			
exercises	weight	reps	time under tension
leg extension			
squat			
dumbbell pullover			
chin-up			
dumbbell fly			
bench press			
biceps curl			
lying leg curl			
calf raise			
abdominal crunch			

9.6 Sample full body workout with post-exhaustion A

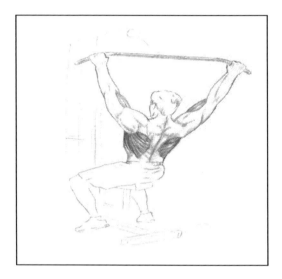

Figure 20: Lat pull-down

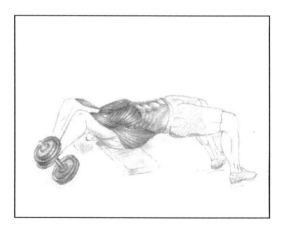

Figure 21: Pullover

Exercises

compound set of incline bench press and pec-deck fly
compound set of leg press and leg extension
compound set of lat pull-down and pullover
biceps curl
leg raise

Date			
exercises	weight	reps	time under tension
incline bench press			
pec-deck fly			
leg press			
leg extension			
lat pull-down			
pullover			
biceps curl			
leg raise			

9.7 Sample full body workout with post-exhaustion B

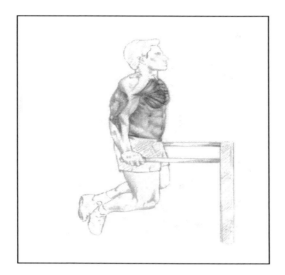

Figure 22: Dips

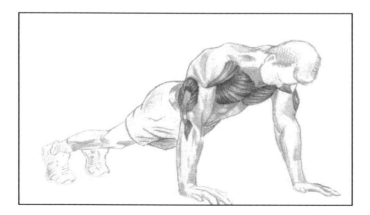

Figure 23: Push-up

Exercises

compound set of squat and leg extension
compound set of lat pull-down and pullover
compound set of dips and push-up
dumbbell curl
abdominal crunch

Date			
exercises	weight	reps	time under tension
squat			
leg extension			
lat-pull-down			
dumbbell pullover			
dips			
push-up			
dumbbell curl			
abdominal crunch			

9.8 Split program: Sample upper/lower body split

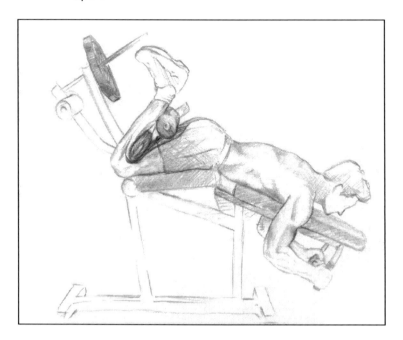

Figure 24: Leg curl

Workout 1

squat
leg extension
leg curl
calf raise
abdominal crunch

Date			
exercises	weight	reps	time under tension
squat			
leg extension			
leg curl			
calf raise			
abdominal crunch			

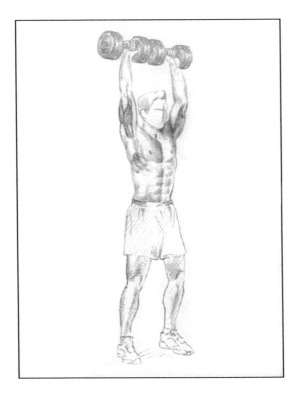

Figure 25: Shoulder press

Workout 2

incline dumbbell press
lat pull-down
shoulder press
dumbbell lateral raise
biceps curl
dips

Date			
exercises	weight	reps	time under tension
incline dumbbell press			
lat pull-down			
shoulder press			
dumbbell lateral raise			
biceps curl			
dips			

9.9   Split program: Sample upper/lower body split with pre-exhaustion

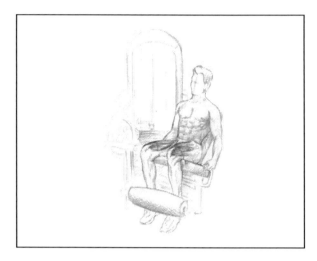

Figure 26: Leg extension

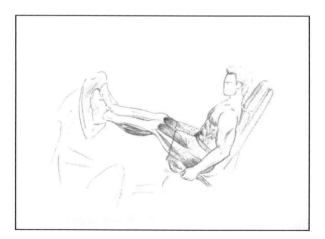

Figure 27: Leg press

Workout 1

compound set of leg extension and leg press
compound set of calf raise and leg curl
compound set of leg raise and abdominal crunch

Date			
exercises	weight	reps	time under tension
leg extension			
leg press			
calf raise			
leg curl			
leg raise			
abdominal crunch			

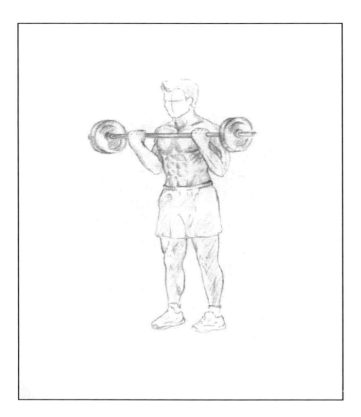

Figure 28: Biceps curl

Workout 2

compound set of incline dumbbell fly and incline bench press
compound set of lat pullover and back row
compound set of dumbbell lateral raise and shoulder press
biceps curl
triceps kick-back

Date			
exercises	weight	reps	time under tension
incline dumbbell fly			
incline bench press			
lat pullover			
back row			
dumbbell lateral raise			
shoulder press			
biceps curl			
triceps kick-back			

9.10 Split program: Sample upper/lower body split with post-exhaustion

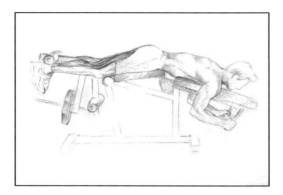

Figure 29: Leg curl

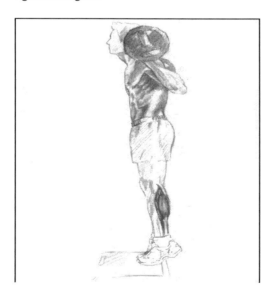

Figure 30: Calf raise

Workout 1

compound set of squat and leg extension
compound set of leg curl and calf raise
compound set of leg raise and abdominal crunch

Date			
exercises	weight	reps	time under tension
squat			
leg extension			
leg curl			
calf raise			
leg raise			
abdominal crunch			

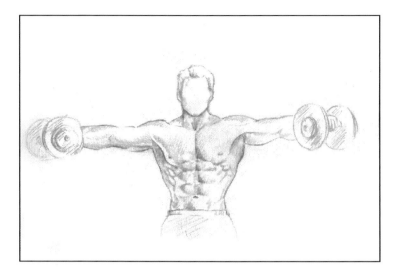

Figure 31: Dumbbell lateral raise

Workout 2

compound set of bench press and push-up
compound set of lat pull-down and pullover
compound set of shoulder press and dumbbell lateral raise
biceps curl
triceps extension

Date			
exercises	weight	reps	time under tension
bench press			
push-up			
lat pull-down			
pullover			
shoulder press			
dumbbell lateral raise			
biceps curl			
triceps extension			

9.11   Split program: Push-pull split A (two-way split)

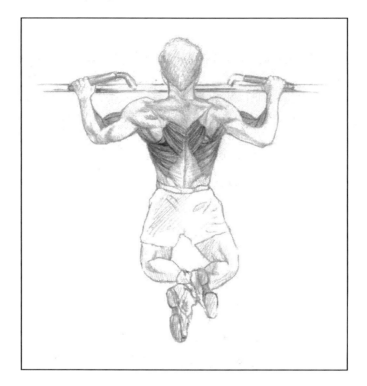

Figure 32: Chin-up

Workout 1

Legs, back, and biceps

deadlift
leg press
chin-up
pullover
shrug
preacher curl
dumbbell hammer curl

Date			
exercises	weight	reps	time under tension
deadlift			
leg press			
chin-up			
pullover			
shrug			
preacher curl			
dumbbell hammer curl			

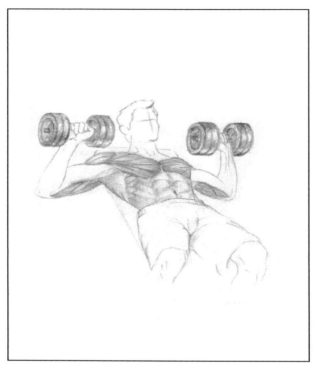

Figure 33: Incline dumbbell press

Workout 2

Chest, shoulders, and triceps

bench press
incline dumbbell press
dumbbell lateral raise
shoulder press
dips
triceps extension
abdominal crunch

Date			
exercises	weight	reps	time under tension
bench press			
incline dumbbell press			
dumbbell lateral raise			
shoulder press			
dips			
triceps extension			
abdominal crunch			

9.12 Split program: Push-pull split B (three-way split)

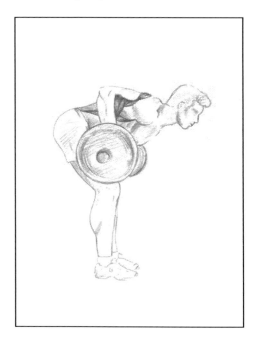

Figure 34: Back row

Workout 1

Back and biceps

back row
lat pull-down
pullover
shrug
alternate dumbbell hammer curl
preacher curl

Date			
exercises	weight	reps	time under tension
back row			
lat pull-down			
pullover			
shrug			
alternate dumbbell hammer curl			
preacher curl			

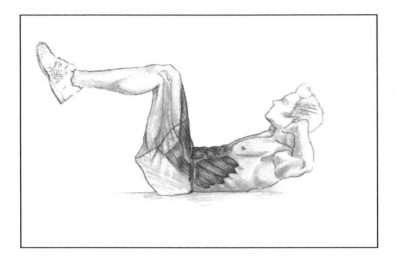

Figure 35: Abdominal crunch

Workout 2

Legs and abdominals

leg press
leg extension
leg curl
front squat
calf raise
abdominal crunch

Date			
exercises	weight	reps	time under tension
leg press			
leg extension			
leg curl			
front squat			
calf raise			
abdominal crunch			

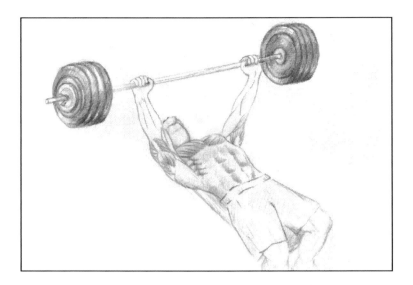

Figure 36: Incline bench press

Workout 3

Chest, shoulders, and triceps

incline bench press
flat bench dumbbell press
shoulder press
dumbbell lateral raise
dips
triceps kick-back

Date			
exercises	weight	reps	time under tension
incline bench press			
flat bench dumbbell press			
shoulder press			
dumbbell lateral raise			
dips			
triceps kick-backs			

These training programs are examples that have proven to work very well. If for some reason, you cannot do a certain exercise, you can replace it with a similar one. This is absolutely okay as long as you stick to the basic guidelines of High Intensity Training. After all, the aim of all this is to find a program that works well for you.

10   Intensity and consistency

Some people might have doubts about the concept of high intensity training. We have heard many times over that more is always better, that more training will produce better results and that *three* is the ideal number of sets to perform for each exercise to achieve optimum results.

Despite what some muscle magazines tell us, High Intensity Training is not just another training method among several. It is a practical application of training science. These magazines are published monthly and must come up with something new as often as possible to entertain their readers on a regular basis. However, when it comes to training there is nothing new. The way the human body adapts to imposed stimuli has not changed in thousand years. Training methods are not the same as fashion trends although they are sometimes "hyped" in a similar way. To be successful, training needs to provide the body with an adequate stimulus (i.e. intensity must be high enough) followed by enough rest and recuperation to let the corresponding adaptive processes take place. Adequate rest is not less important than the training stimulus itself.

It is true that to become an outstanding football player it is not enough to practice intensively twice a week for 60 minutes. Neither will two or three intense sessions on the basketball court be enough to make it to the NBA. These sports require skill sets that take much time to acquire. To set a new world record in weightlifting you will have to repeat your lift many times and it may take years to develop perfect lifting technique. Beginner weightlifters often practice with an unloaded bar or even a broomstick for several months. After months of training (or rather, practice), they add weight and continue training progressively.

Despite of what we read in some magazines, training for hours each day is neither necessary nor sensible for developing a strong, lean, healthy and very muscular physique. For most it is even counterproductive. Even if multiple-set training produced a few per cent more strength and muscle mass than High Intensity Training (which it does not), would this justify training three times as much?

Those who are considering a three-set training program should ask themselves if they would work three times as much in their jobs, spending three times as many hours for the prospect of a few percent more pay. We are talking about 120 hours a week instead of 40. Even if a double-split training program six days a week was ideal (which it is not) for improving strength and body composition as some muscle magazines claim, how many people have the time to work out twelve times per week? Not to mention the ability to regenerate. Could they continue such a kind of training over a long period of time?

After all, for most people *consistency* is a deciding factor for a successful training program: Finding the kind of training that you can perform under realistic conditions for as long as you want, ideally for the rest of your life. A kind of training that is safe, efficient, and healthy. A kind of training that does not require expensive food supplements or even drugs for the body to fully recover between workouts. A kind of training that effectively triggers physiological adaptations in terms of muscle hypertrophy and increasing strength.

This is exactly what High Intensity Training is.

Recommended Reading

Taleb, Nassim Nicolas (2012). *Antifragile. Things that gain from Disorder*. New York: Random House.

McGuff, Doug & Little, John (2009). *Body by Science. A research-based program for strength training, body building, and complete fitness in 12 minutes a week*. New York: McGraw-Hill.

Zimbardo, Philip & Boyd, John (2008). *The Time Paradox. Using the New Psychology to Your Advantage*. London: Simon & Schuster.

Carpinelli, Ralph (2002). Berger in retrospect: effect of varied weight-training programmes on strength. *British Journal of Sports Medicine, 36* (5), 319-324.

Fisher, James, Steele, James & Smith, Dave (2013). Evidence-based resistance training recommendations for muscular hypertrophy. *Medicina Sportiva, 17* (4), 217-235.

Endnotes

Endnotes

[1] Zimbardo, P. & Boyd, J. (2008). *The Time Paradox. Using the New Psychology to Your Advantage*. London: Simon & Schuster.

[2] Taleb, N.N. (2012). *Antifragile. Things that gain from Disorder*. New York: Random House.

[3] Jones, A. (1970). *Nautilus Bulletin No. 1*. http://baye.com/wp-content/uploads/2011/01/Nautilus-Training-Principles-Bulletin-1.pdf, Accessed June 18, 2015.

[4] Darden, E. (2004). *The New High Intensity Training*. Emmaus: Rodale Books.

[5] Roach, R. (2011). *Muscle, Smoke & Mirrors*. Bloomington: Author House.

[6] Jones, A. *Nautilus Bulletin No. 3*. Unpublished.

[7] Berger, R.A. (1962). Effect of varied weight training programs on strength. *Research Quarterly, 33* (2), 168-181.

[8] Carpinelli, R. (2002). Berger in retrospect: effect of varied weight-training programmes on strength. *British Journal of Sports Medicine, 36* (5), 319-324.

[9] Berger, R.A. (1963). Comparative effects of three weight training programs. *Research Quarterly, 34* (3), 396-398.

[10] Berger, R.A. (1965). Application of research findings in progressive resistance exercise to physical therapy. *Journal of the Association of Physical and Mental Rehabilitation, 19* (6), 200-203.

[11] Berger, R.A. (1972). Effect of varied sets of static training on dynamic strength. *American Corrective Therapy Journal, 26* (2), 52-54.

[12] Berger, R.A. (1972). Strength improvement. *Strength and Health, 44-45*, 70-71.

[13] Berger, R.A. (1973). *Conditioning for men*. Boston: Allyn and Bacon.

[14] Berger, R.A. (1984). *Introduction to weight training*. Englewood Cliffs, NJ: Prentice-Hall.

[15] http://www.bodybuilding.com/fun/cyberpump8.htm, Accessed June 18, 2015.

[16] Rhea, M.R., Alvar, B.A. & Burkett, L.N. (2002). Single versus multiple sets for strength: a meta-analysis to address the controversy. *Research Quarterly for Exercise and Sport, 73* (4), 485-488.

[17] Rhea, M.R., Alvar, B.A., Burkett, L.N. & Ball, S.D. (2003). A Meta-analysis to determine the Dose Response for Strength Development. *Medicine and Science in Sports and Exercise, 35* (3), 456-464.

[18] Peterson M.D., Rhea M.R. & Alvar, B.A. (2004) Maximizing strength development in athletes: a meta-analysis to determine the dose-response relationship. *Journal of Strength and Conditioning Research, 18* (2), 377-382.

[19] Wolfe, B.L., LeMura, L. M. & Cole, P. J. (2004). Quantitative analysis of single vs. multiple-set programs in resistance training. *Journal of Strength and Conditioning Research, 18* (1), 35-47.

[20] National Strength and Conditioning Association (2005). Session Review: The end of the single-set versus multiple-set discussion. *NSCA Bulletin, 26*, 7.

[21] Giessing, J. & Eichmann, B. (2012). *Muscle hypertrophy and strength increases after ten weeks of high intensity training (HIT)*. Marburg: Tectum.

[22] Carpinelli, R. (2002). Berger in retrospect: effect of varied weight-training programmes on strength. *British Journal of Sports Medicine, 36* (5), 322.

[23] Fisher, J., Steele, J. & Smith, D. (2013). Evidence-based resistance training recommendations for muscular hypertrophy. *Medicina Sportiva, 17* (4), 217-235.

[24] Schwarzenegger, A. (2012). *Total Recall. My unbelievably true life story*. London: Simon & Schuster.

[25] Fleck, S.J. & Kraemer, W.J. (1987). *Designing resistance training programs*. Champaign, IL: Human Kinetics.

[26] Best, M. & Neuhauser, D. (2004). Ignaz Semmelweis and the birth of infection control. *Quality and Safety in Health Care, 13* (3), 233-234.

[27] Simpson, G.G. (1943). Mammals and the Nature of Continents. *American Journal of Science*, *241* (1), 1-31.

[28] Fleck, S.J. & Kraemer, W.J. (2014). *Designing resistance training programs*. Champaign, IL: Human Kinetics.

[29] Fleck, S.J. & Kraemer, W.J. (2014). *Designing resistance training programs*. Champaign, IL: Human Kinetics.

[30] Giessing, J., Fisher, J., Steele, J., Rothe, F., Raubold, K. & Eichmann, B. (2014). The effects of low volume resistance training with and without advanced techniques in trained participants. *Journal of Sports Medicine and Physical Fitness*, *54*, 1-22.

[31] Mentzer, M. (1992). Is there really a science of bodybuilding? *Flex*, *10*, 34-36, 70, 156.

[32] Schlumberger, A. & Schmidtbleicher, D. (1999): Einsatz-Training als trainingsmethodische Alternative – Möglichkeiten und Grenzen. *Leistungssport*, *29* (3), 9-11.

[33] Schwarzenegger, A. (1997). How I built my enormous delts. Musclemag: Portrait of an icon, 30-37.

[34] Schwarzenegger, A. (1997). How I built my massive 22.5-inch arms. Musclemag: Portrait of an icon, 82-93.

[35] Jones, A. (1972). Bodybuilding as I have seen it...as I see it now. *Muscle Training Illustrated*, http://www.arthurjonesexercise.com/MuscleTraining/Body1.PDF, Accessed June 18, 2015.

References and related studies

American College of Sports Medicine (2013). *ACSM's Resource Manual for Guidelines for Exercise Testing and Prescription* (7th edition). Baltimore, MD: Lippincott Williams and Wilkins.

Atha, J. (1981). Strengthening muscle. *Exercise and Sport Sciences Reviews, 9*, 1-73.

Baechle, T.R. (1994). *Essentials of Training and Conditioning*. Champaign, IL: Human Kinetics.

Baker, J.S., Davies, B., Cooper, S.M., Wong, D.P., Buchan, D.S. & Kilgore, L. (2013). Strength and Body Composition Changes in Recreationally Strength-Trained Individuals: Comparison of One versus Three Sets Resistance-Training Programmes. *BioMed Research International*. http://dx.doi.org/10.1155/2013/615901, Accessed June 18, 2015.

Becque, M.D., Lochmann J.D. & Melrose, D.R. (2000). Effects of oral creatine supplementation on muscular strength and body composition. *Medicine and Science in Sports and Exercise, 32* (3), 654-658.

Behm D.G. (1995). Neuromuscular implications and applications of resistance training. *Journal of Strength and Conditioning Research, 9* (4), 264-74.

Bemben, D.A., Fetters, N.L., Bemben, M.G., Nabavi, N. & Koh, E.T. (2000). Musculoskeletal responses to high- and low-intensity resistance training in early postmenopausal women. *Medicine and Science in Sports and Exercise, 32* (11), 1949-1957.

Berger, R.A. (1962). Effect of varied weight training programs on strength. *Research Quarterly, 33* (2), 168-181.

Berger, R.A. (1963). Comparative effects of three weight training programs. *Research Quarterly, 34* (3), 396-398.

Berger, R.A. (1965). Application of research findings in progressive resistance exercise to physical therapy. *Journal of the Association of Physical and Mental Rehabilitation, 19* (6), 200-203.

Berger, R.A. (1972). Effect of varied sets of static training on dynamic strength. *American Corrective Therapy Journal, 26* (2), 52-54.

Berger, R.A. (1972). Strength improvement. *Strength and Health*, 44-45, 70-71.

Berger, R.A. (1973). *Conditioning for men*. Boston: Allyn and Bacon.

Berger, R.A. (1982). *Applied exercise physiology*. Philadelphia: Lea & Febiger.

Berger, R.A. (1984). *Introduction to weight training*. Englewood Cliffs, NJ: Prentice-Hall.

Borst, S.E., De Hoyos, D.V., Garzarella, L., Vincent, K., Pollock, B.H., Lowenthal, D.T. & Pollock, M.L. (2001). Effects of resistance training on insulin-like growth factor-I and IGF binding proteins. *Medicine and Science in Sports and Exercise, 33* (4), 648-653.

Bosco, C., Colli, R., Bonomi, R., Von Duvillard, S.P. & Viru, A. (2000). Monitoring strength training: neuromuscular and hormonal profile. *Medicine and Science in Sports and Exercise, 32* (1), 202-208.

Bowers, R.W. & Fox, E.L. (1992). *Sports Physiology*. Dubuque: W.C. Brown Publishers.

Boyer B.T. (1990). A comparison of three strength training programs on women. *Journal of Applied Sports Science Research, 4* (5), 88-94.

Braith, R.W., Graves, J.E., Pollock, M.L., Leggett, S.H., Carpenter, D.M. & Colvin, A.B. (1989). Comparison of two versus three days per week of variable resistance training during 10- and 18-week programs. *International Journal of Sports Medicine, 10* (6), 450-454.

Brenner, M., Rankin, J.W. & Sebolt, D. (2000). The effect of creatine supplementation during resistance training in women. *Journal of Strength and Conditioning Research, 14* (2), 207-213.

Brooks, G.A., Fahey, T.D. & White, T. (1996). Neurons, motor unit recruitment, and integrative control of movement. In G.A. Brooks, T.D. Fahey, & T. White (Eds.), *Exercise Physiology* (pp. 328-359). Mountainview: Mayfield Press.

Bush, J.A., Dohi, K., Mastro, A.M., Volek, J.S., Lynch, J.M., Triplett-McBride, N.T., Putukian, M., Sebastianelli, W.J., Newton, R.U., Hakkinen, K. & Kraemer, W.J. (2000). Exercise and recovery responses of lymphokines to heavy resistance exercise. *Journal of Strength and Conditioning Research, 14* (3), 344-349.

Byrd, R., Chandler, T.J., Conley, M.S., Fry, A.C., Haff, G.G., Koch, A., Hatfield, F., Kirksey, K.B., McBride, J., McBride, T., Newton, H., O'Bryant, H.S., Stone, M.H., Pierce, K.C., Plisk, S., Ritchie-Stone, M. & Wathen, D. (1999). Strength training: single versus multiple sets. *Sports Medicine, 27* (6), 409-416.

Capen, E.K. (1956). Study of four programs of heavy resistance exercise for development of muscular strength. *Research Quarterly, 27* (2), 132-142.

Carpinelli, R.N. & Otto R.M. (1998). Strength training. Single versus multiple sets. *Sports Medicine, 26* (2), 73-84.

Chestnut, J.L. & Docherty, D. (1999). The effects of 4 and 10 repetition maximum weight-training protocols on neuromuscular adaptations in untrained men. *Journal of Strength and Conditioning Research, 13* (4), 353-359.

Ciriello, V.M., Holden, W.L. & Evans, W.J. (1982). The effects of two isokinetic training regimens on muscle strength and fiber composition. In H.G. Knuttgen, J.A. Vogel & J. Poortmans (Eds.), *Biochemistry of exercise* (pp. 787-793). Champaign, IL: Human Kinetics.

Clarke, D.H. (1973). Adaptations in strength and muscular endurance resulting from exercise. *Exercise and Sport Sciences Reviews, 1,* 73-102.

Coleman, A.E. (1977). Nautilus vs. Universal Gym strength training in adult males. *American Corrective Therapy Journal, 31* (4), 103-107.

Curto, M.A. & Fisher, M.M. (1999). The effect of single vs. multiple sets of resistance exercise on strength in trained males. *Medicine and Science in Sports and Exercise, 31,* 114.

Darden E. (1978). Strength training principles. In J.A. Peterson (Ed.), *Total fitness: the Nautilus way* (pp. 157-174). West Point, NY: Leisure Press.

De Hoyos, D.V., Abe T., Garzarella, L., Hass, C., Nordman, M. & Pollock, M. (1998). Effects of 6 months of high- or low-volume resistance training on muscular strength and endurance. *Medicine and Science in Sports and Exercise, 30* (5), 165.

De Hoyos, D.V., Herring, D., Garzarella, L., Werber, G., Brechue, W.F. & Pollock, M. L. (1997). Effect of strength training volume on the development of strength and power in adolescent tennis players. *Medicine and Science in Sports and Exercise, 29* (5), 164.

De Vries, H.A. & Housh, T.J. (1994). *Physiology of exercise for physical education, athletics, and sports science.* Madison: Brown & Benchmark.

Di Nubile, N.A. (1991). Strength training. *Clinics in Sports Medicine, 10* (1), 33-62.

Dudley, G.A., Tesch, P.A., Miller, M.A. & Buchanan, M.D. (1991). Importance of eccentric actions in performance adaptations to resistance training. *Aviation, Space, and Environmental Medicine, 62* (6), 543-550.

Enoka, R.M. (1988). Chronic adaptations. In R.M. Enoka (Ed.), *Neuromechanical basis of kinesiology* (pp. 303-349). Champaign, IL: Human Kinetics.

Fahey, T.D. (1989). *Basic Weight Training*. Mountainview: Mayfield Press.

Feigenbaum, M.S. & Pollock, M.L. (1997). Strength training: rationale for current guidelines for adult fitness programs. *Physician and Sportsmedicine, 25* (2), 44-64.

Feigenbaum, M.S. & Pollock, M.L. (1999). Prescription of resistance training for health and disease. *Medicine and Science in Sports and Exercise, 31* (1), 38-45.

Fiatarone, M.A., O'Neill, E.F., Ryan, N.D., Clements, K.M., Solares, G.R., Nelson, M.E., Roberts, S.B., Kehayias, J.J., Lipsitz, L.A. & Evans, W.J. (1994). Exercise training and nutritional supplementation for physical frailty in very elderly people. *New England Journal of Medicine, 330*, 1769-75.

Fincher, G.E. (2000). The effect of high intensity resistance training on peak upper and lower body power among collegiate football players. *Medicine and Science in Sports and Exercise, 32* (5), 657.

Fleck, S.J. (1999). Periodized strength training: a critical review. *Journal of Strength and Conditioning Research, 13* (1), 82-89.

Fleck, S.J. & Kraemer, W.J. (1987). *Designing resistance training programs*. Champaign, IL: Human Kinetics.

Fleck, S.J. & Kraemer, W.J. (1988). Resistance training: basic principles (part 1 of 4). *Physician and Sportsmedicine, 16* (3), 160-71.

Fleck, S.J. & Kraemer, W.J. (1996). *Periodization breakthrough!* Ronkonkoma, NY: Advanced Research Press.

Fleck, S.J. & Kraemer, W.J. (1997). *Designing resistance training programs* (2nd edition). Champaign, IL: Human Kinetics.

Fox, E.L. (1979). *Sports Physiology*. Philadelphia: Saunders.

Fox, E.L., Bowers, R.W. & Foss, M.L. (1993). Development of muscular strength, endurance, and flexibility. In E.L. Fox, R.W. Bowers & M.L. Foss (Eds.), *The physiological basis for exercise and sport* (pp. 158-192). Madison, WI: Brown & Benchmark Publishers.

Fox, E.L. & Mathews, D.K. (1981). *The physiological basis of physical education and athletics*. Philadelphia: Saunders.

Fry, A.C., Webber, J.M., Weiss, L.W., Fry, M.D. & Li, Y. (2000). Impaired performances with excessive high-intensity free-weight training. *Journal of Strength and Conditioning Research, 14* (1), 54-61.

Garhammer, J. (1981). Equipment for the development of athletic strength and power. *National Strength and Conditioning Association Journal, 3*, 24-26.

Garhammer, J. (1987). *Sports Illustrated Strength Training*. New York: Time.

Garhammer, J. & Takano, B. (1992). Training for weightlifting. In P.V. Komi (Ed.), *Strength and Power in Sport* (pp. 357-369). Oxford: Blackwell Scientific Publications.

Girouard, C.K. & Hurley, B.F. (1995). Does strength training inhibit gains in range of motion from flexibility training in older adults? *Medicine and Science in Sports and Exercise, 27*, 1444-1449.

Gravelle, B.L. & Blessing, D.L. (2000). Physiological adaptation in women concurrently training for strength and endurance. *Journal of Strength and Conditioning Research, 14* (1), 5-13.

Graves, J.E., Holmes, B.L., Leggett, S.H., Carpenter, D.M. & Pollock, M.L. (1991). *Single versus multiple set dynamic and isometric lumbar extension training*. Eleventh International Congress of the World Confederation for Physical Therapy. Proceedings Book III, Great Britain (pp. 1340-1342).

Guyton, A.C. (1991). *Textbook of Medical Physiology* (8th edition). Philadelphia: Elsevier.

Guyton, A.C. & Hall, J.E. (1996). *Textbook of Medical Physiology* (11th edition). Philadelphia: Elsevier.

Hakkinen, K. & Komi, P.V. (1983). Electromyographic changes during strength training and detraining. *Medicine and Science in Sports and Exercise, 15* (6), 455-460.

Hakkinen, K., Komi, P.V. & Kauhanen, H. (1987). EMG, muscle fiber, and force production characteristics during a 1-year training period in elite weight lifters. *European Journal of Applied Physiology, 56*, 419-427.

Hakkinen, K., Pakarinen, A., Alen, M., Kauhanen, H. & Komi, P.V. (1988). Neuromuscular and hormonal adaptations in athletes to strength training in two years. *Journal of Applied Physiology, 65* (6), 2406-2412.

Harris, G.R., Stone, M.H., O'Bryant, H.S., Proulx, C.M. & Johnson, R.L. (2000). Short term performance effects of high power, high force, or combined weight-training methods. *Journal of Strength and Conditioning Research*, *14* (1), 14-20.

Hass, C.J., Garzarella, L., De Hoyos, D.V. & Pollock, M.L. (1998). Effects of training volume on strength and endurance in experienced resistance trained adults. *Medicine and Science in Sports and Exercise*, *30* (5), 115.

Hass, C.J., Garzarella, L., De Hoyos, D. & Pollock, M.L. (2000). Single versus multiple sets in long-term recreational weightlifters. *Medicine and Science in Sports and Exercise*, *32* (1), 235-242.

Hatfield, F.C. (1989). *Power: A scientific approach*. Chicago: Contemporary Books.

Hisaeda, H., Miyagawa, K., Kuno, S., Fukunaga, T. & Muraoka, I. (1996). Influence of two different modes of resistance training in female subjects. *Ergonomics*, *39* (6), 842-852.

Howley, E.T. & Franks, B.D. (1986). *Health Fitness Instructor's Handbook*. Champaign, IL: Human Kinetics.

Hurley, B.F., Redmond, R.A., Pratley, R.E., Treuth, M.S., Rogers, M.A & Goldberg, A.P. (1995). Effects of strength training on muscle hypertrophy and muscle cell distribution in older men. *International Journal of Sports Medicine*, *16* (6), 378-384.

Jacobson, B.H. (1986). A comparison of two progressive weight training techniques on knee extensor strength. *Athletic Training*, *21* (4), 315-318, 390.

Jesse, C., McGee, J., Gibson, J., Stone, M. & Williams, J. (1988). A comparison of Nautilus and free weight training. *Journal of Applied Sports Science Research*, *2* (3), 59.

Jones, A. (1978). Flexibility as a result of exercise. In J.A. Peterson (Ed.), *Total fitness: the Nautilus way* (pp. 134-141). West Point, NY: Leisure Press.

Kelley, G.A. & Kelley, K.S. (2000). Progressive resistance exercise and resting blood pressure. A meta-analysis of randomized controlled trials. *Hypertension*, *35* (3), 838-843.

Knuttgen, H.G. (1976). Development of muscular strength and endurance. In H.G. Knuttgen (Ed.), *Neuromuscular mechanisms for therapeutic and conditioning exercise* (pp. 97-118). Baltimore: University Park Press.

Koffler, K.H., Menkes, A., Redmond, R.A., Whitehead, W.E., Pratley, R.E. & Hurley, B.F. (1992). Strength training accelerates gastrointestinal transit in middle-aged and older men. *Medicine and Science in Sports and Exercise*, *24*, 415-419.

Kosmahl, E.M., Mackarey, P.J. & Buntz, S.E. (1989). Nautilus training system versus traditional weight training system. *Journal of Orthopaedic and Sports Physical Therapy*, *11*, 253-258.

Kraemer, W.J. (1997). A series of studies-the physiological basis for strength training in American football: fact over philosophy. *Journal of Strength and Conditioning Research*, *11*, 131-142.

Kraemer, W.J. & Baechle, T.R. (1989). Development of a strength training program. In F.L. Allman & A.J. Ryan (Eds.), *Sports Medicine* (pp. 113-127). Orlando: Academic Press.

Kraemer, W.J., Duncan, N.D. & Volek, J.S. (1998). Resistance training and elite athletes: Adaptations and program considerations. *Journal of Orthopaedic and Sports Physical Therapy*, *28* (2), 110-119.

Kraemer, W.J. & Fleck, S.J. (1988). Resistance training: exercise prescription (part 4 of 4). *Physician and Sportsmedicine*, *16* (6), 69-81.

Kraemer, W.J., Fleck, S.J. & Deschenes, M. (1988). A review: factors in exercise prescription of resistance training. *National Strength and Conditioning Association Journal*, *10* (5), 36-41.

Kraemer, W.J., Fleck, S.J. & Evans, W.J. (1996). Strength and power training: physiological mechanisms of adaptation. *Exercise and Sport Sciences Reviews*, *24*, 363-397.

Kraemer, W.J. & Koziris, L.P. (1992). Muscle strength training: techniques and considerations. *Physiotherapy Theory and Practice*, *2* (1), 54-68.

Kraemer, W.J. & Koziris, L.P. (1994). Olympic weightlifting and powerlifting. In D.R. Lamb, H.G. Knuttgen & R. Murray (Eds.), *Physiology and Nutrition for Competitive Sport* (pp. 1-54). Carmel: Cooper.

Kraemer, W.J., Newton, R.V., Bush, J., Volek, J., Triplett, N.T. & Koziris, L.P. (1995). Varied multiple set resistance training programs produce greater gains than single set program. *Medicine and Science in Sports and Exercise*, *27* (5), 195.

Kraemer, W.J., Ratamess, N., Fry, A.C., Triplett-McBride, T., Koziris, L.P., Bauer, J.A., Lynch, J.M. & Fleck, S.J. (2000). Influence of resistance training volume and periodization on physiological and performance adaptations in collegiate women tennis players. *American Journal of Sports Medicine*, *28* (5), 626-633.

Kramer, J.B., Stone, M S., O'Bryant, H.S., Conley, M.S., Johnson, R.L., Nieman, D.C., Honeycutt, D.R. & Hoke, T.P. (1997). Effect of single vs. multiple sets of weight training: impact of volume, intensity, and variation. *Journal of Strength and Conditioning Research, 11* (3), 143-147.

Krieger, J.W. (2010). Single vs. multiple sets of resistance exercise for muscle hypertrophy: a meta-analysis. *Journal of Strength and Conditioning Research, 24* (4), 1150-1159.

Lamb, D.R. (1984). *Physiology of Exercise, Responses and Adaptations.* New York: Macmillan.

Larshus, J.L., Hoeger, W.K. & Moore, J.R. (1997). Effects of multiple exercise training on the development of tricep strength. *Research Quarterly for Exercise and Sport,* 33-4.

Leighton, J.R., Holmes, D., Benson, J., Wooten, B. & Schmerer, R. (1967). A study of the effectiveness of ten different methods of progressive resistance exercise on the development of strength, flexibility, girth and bodyweight. *Journal of the Association of Physical and Mental Rehabilitation, 21,* 78-81.

Lemmer, J.T., Ivey, F.M., Ryan, A.S., Martel, G.F., Hurlbut, D.E., Metter, J.E., Fozard, J.L., Fleg, J.L. & Hurley, B.F. (2001). Effect of strength training on resting metabolic rate and physical activity: age and gender comparisons. *Medicine and Science in Sports and Exercise, 33* (4), 532-541.

Liederman, E. (1925). Quality of muscle the basis of strength. In E. Liederman (Ed.), *Secrets of strength* (pp. 116-130). New York, NY: Earle Liederman.

Lillegard, W.A. & Terrio, J.D. (1994). Appropriate strength training. *Medical Clinics of North America, 78* (2), 457-77.

Luecke, T., Wendeln, H., Campos, G.R., Hagerman, F.C., Hikida, R.S. & Staron, R.S. (1998). The effects of three different resistance training programs on cardiorespiratory function. *Medicine and Science in Sports and Exercise, 30* (5), 1125.

Martel, G.F., Horblut, D.E., Lott, M.E., Lemmer, J.T., Ivey, F.M., Roth, S.M., Rogers, M.A., Fleg, J.L. & Hurley, B.F. (1999). Strength training normalizes resting blood pressure in 65- to 73-year-old men and women with high normal blood pressure. *Journal of the American Geriatrics Society, 47* (10), 1215-1221.

Marx, J.O., Ratamess, N.A., Nindl, B.C., Gotshalk, L.A., Volek, J.S., Dohi, K., Bush, J.A., Gómez, A.L., Mazzetti, S.A., Fleck, S.J., Häkkinen, K., Newton, R.U. & Kraemer, W.J. (2001). Low-volume circuit versus high-volume periodized resistance training in women. *Medicine and Science in Sports and Exercise, 33* (4), 635-643.

Mazzetti, S.A., Kraemer, W.J., Volek, J.S., Duncan, N.D., Ratamess, N.A., Gómez, A.L., Newton, R.U., Häkkinen, K. & Fleck, S.J. (2000). The influence of direct supervision of resistance training on strength performance. *Medicine and Science in Sports and Exercise, 32* (6), 1175-1184.

McArdle, W.D., Katch, F.I. & Katch, V.L. (1996). *Exercise Physiology: Energy, Nutrition, and Human Performance* (4th edition). Baltimore: Williams & Wilkins.

McArdle, W.D., Katch, F.I. & Katch, V.L. (1996). Muscular strength: training muscles to become stronger. In *Exercise physiology: energy, nutrition, and human performance* (pp. 417-455). Baltimore, MD: Williams & Wilkins.

McCartney, N., McKelvie, R.S., Martin, J., Sale, D.G. & MacDougall, J.D. (1993). Weight-training induced attenuation of the circulatory response to weightlifting in older men. *Journal of Applied Physiology, 74* (3), 1056-1060.

McDonagh, M.N. & Davies, C.M. (1984). Adaptive response of mammalian skeletal muscle to exercise with high loads. *European Journal of Applied Physiology, 52*, 139-155.

Menkes, A., Mazel, S., Redmond, R.A., Koffler, K., Libanati, C.R., Gundberg, C.M., Zizic, T.M., Hagberg, J.M., Pratley, R.E. & Hurley, B.F. (1993). Strength training increases regional bone mineral density and bone remodeling in middle-aged and older men. *Journal of Applied Physiology, 74* (5), 2478-2484.

Messier, S.P. & Dill, M.E. (1985). Alterations in strength and maximal oxygen uptake consequent to Nautilus circuit weight training. *Research Quarterly for Exercise and Sport, 56* (4), 345-351.

Miller, J.P., Pratley, R.E., Goldberg, A.P., Gordon, P., Rubin, M., Treuth, M.S., Ryan, A.S. & Hurley, B.F. (1994). Strength training increases insulin action in healthy 50- to 65-year-old men. *Journal of Applied Physiology, 77* (3), 1122-1127.

Moffatt, R.J. & Cucuzzo, N. (1993). Strength considerations for exercise prescription. In *Resource Manual Guidelines for Exercise Testing and Prescription* (pp. 337-343). Philadelphia: Lea and Febiger.

Moran, G. & McGlynn, G. (2001). *Dynamics of Strength Training.* New York: McGraw-Hill.

National Strength and Conditioning Association (2005). Session Review: The end of the single-set versus multiple-set discussion. *NSCA Bulletin, 26*, 7.

Nicklas, B.J., Ryan, A.J., Treuth, M.M., Harman, S.M., Blackman, M.R., Hurley, B.F. & Rogers, M.A. (1995). Testosterone, growth hormone and IGF-I responses to acute and chronic resistive exercise in men aged 55-70 years. *International Journal of Sports Medicine, 16* (7), 445-450.

Ostrowski, K.J., Wilson, G.J., Weatherby, R., Murphy, P.W. & Lyttle, A.D. (1997). The effect of weight training volume on hormonal output and muscular size and function. *Journal of Strength and Conditioning Research, 11* (3), 148-154.

Parker, N.D., Hunter, G.R., Treuth, M.S., Kekes-Szabo, T., Kell, S.H., Weinsier, R. & White, M. (1996). Effects of strength training on cardiovascular responses during a submaximal walk and a weight-loaded walking test in older females. *Journal of Cardiopulmonary Rehabilitation, 16* (1), 56-62.

Peterson, M.D., Rhea, M.R. & Alvar, B.A. (2004). Maximizing strength development in athletes: a meta-analysis to determine the dose-response relationship. *Journal of Strength and Conditioning Research, 18* (2), 377-382.

Plowman, S.A. & Smith, D.L. (1997). *Exercise physiology for health, fitness, and performance*. Baltimore: Lippincott Williams & Wilkins.

Pollock, M.L. (1988). Prescribing exercise for fitness and adherence. In R.K. Dishman (Ed.), *Exercise Adherence: Its Impacts on Public Health* (pp. 259-277). Champaign, IL: Human Kinetics.

Pollock, M.L., Abe, T., De Hoyos, D.V., Garzarella, L., Hass, C.J. & Werber, J. (1998). Muscular hypertrophy responses to 6 months of high- or low-volume resistance training. *Medicine and Science in Sports and Exercise, 30*, 116.

Pollock, M.H., Graves, J.E., Bamman, M.M., Leggett, S.H., Carpenter, D.M., Carr, C., Cirulli, J., Matkozich, J. & Fulton, M. (1993). Frequency and volume of resistance training: effect on cervical extension strength. *Archives of Physical Medicine and Rehabilitation, 74*, 1080-1086.

Pollock, M.L. & Wilmore, J.H. (1990). *Exercise in Health and Disease* (2nd edition). Philadelphia: Saunders.

Powers, S.K. & Howley, E.T. (1997). *Exercise physiology: Theory and Application to Fitness and Performance*. Dubuque: W.C. Brown.

Pratley, R., Nicklas, B., Rubin, M., Miller, J., Smith, A., Smith, M., Hurley, B. & Goldberg, A. (1994). Strength training increases resting metabolic rate and norepinephrine levels in healthy 50-65-year old men. *Journal of Applied Physiology*, *76* (1), 133-137.

Reid, C.M., Yeater, R.A. & Ullrich, I.H. (1987). Weight training and strength, cardiorespiratory functioning and body composition. *British Journal of Sports Medicine*, *21* (1), 40-44.

Rhea, M.R., Alvar, B.A., Ball, S.D. & Burkett, L.N. (2002). Three sets of weight training superior to 1 set with equal intensity for eliciting strength. *Journal of Strength and Conditioning Research*, *16* (4), 525-529.

Rhea, M.R., Alvar, B.A. & Burkett, L.N. (2002). Single versus multiple sets for strength: a meta-analysis to address the controversy. *Research Quarterly for Exercise and Sport*, *73*, 485-488.

Rhea, M.R., Alvar, B.A., Burkett, L.N. & Ball, S.D. (2003). A Meta-analysis to determine the Dose Response for Strength Development. *Medicine and Science in Sports and Exercise*, *35* (3), 456-464.

Rhea, P.L., Ryan, A.S., Nicklas, B., Gordon, P.L., Tracy, B.L., Graham, W., Pratley, R.E., Goldbert, A.P. & Hurley, B.F. (1999). Effects of strength training with and without weight loss on lipoprotein-lipid levels in postmenopausal women. *Clinical Exercise Physiology*, *1* (3), 138-144.

Riley, D.P. (1977). How to organize a strength training program. In *Strength training by the experts* (pp. 97-107). West Point, NY: Leisure Press.

Rooney, K.J., Herbert, R.D. & Balnave, R.J. (1994). Fatigue contributes to the strength training stimulus. *Medicine and Science in Sports and Exercise*, *26* (9), 1160-1164.

Rowles, M.P., Barnard, K.L., Adams, K.J., Berning, J., Kaelin, M., Shimp-Bowerman, J., Denny, D.M. & Swank, A.M. (2000). Single vs. multiple set strength training in male phase II cardiac patients. *Medicine and Science in Sports and Exercise*, *32* (suppl), S91.

Rubin, M.A., Miller, J.P., Ryan, A.S., Treuth, M.S., Patterson, K.Y., Pratley, R.E., Hurley, B.F., Veillon, C., Moser-Veillon, P.B. & Anderson, R.A. (1998). Acute and chronic resistive exercise increase urinary chromium excretion in men as measured with an enriched chromium stable isotope. *Journal of Nutrition*, *128* (1), 73-78.

Ryan, A.S., Hurlbut, D.E., Lott, M.E., Ivey, F.M., Fleg, J., Hurley, B.F. & Goldberg, A.P. (2001). Insulin action after resistive training in insulin resistant older men and women. *Journal of the American Geriatrics Society, 49* (3), 247-253.

Ryan, A.S., Pratley, R.E., Elahi, D. & Goldberg, A.P. (1995). Resistive training increases fat-free mass and maintains RMR despite weight loss in postmenopausal women. *Journal of Applied Physiology, 79* (3), 818-823.

Ryan, A.S., Pratley, R.E., Elahi, D. & Goldberg, A.P. (2000). Changes in plasma leptin and insulin action with resistive training in post-menopausal women. *International Journal of Obesity, 24* (1), 27-32.

Ryan, A.S., Treuth, M.S., Rubin, M.A., Miller, J.P., Nicklas, B.J., Landis, D.M., Pratley, R.E., Libanati, C.R., Gundberg, C.M. & Hurley, B.F. (1994). Effects of strength training on bone mineral density: Hormonal and bone turnover relationships. *Journal of Applied Physiology, 77* (4), 1678-1684.

Sale, D.G. (1987). Influence of exercise and training on motor unit activation. *Exercise and Sport Sciences Reviews, 15,* 95-151.

Sale, D.G. (1988). Neural adaptations to resistance training. *Medicine and Science in Sports and Exercise, 20* (5), 135-145.

Sale, D.G. (1992). Neural adaptation to strength training. In P.V. Komi (Ed.), *Strength and power in sport* (pp. 249-265). Oxford: Blackwell Scientific Publications.

Sanborn, K., Boros, R., Hruby, J., Schilling, B., O'Bryant, H.S., Johnson, R.L., Hoke, T., Stone, M.E. & Stone, M.H. (2000). Short-term performance effects of weight training with multiple sets not to failure vs. a single set to failure in women. *Journal of Strength and Conditioning Research, 14* (3), 328-331.

Schmidtbleicher, D. & Buehrle, M. (1987). Neuronal adaptation and increase of cross-sectional area studying different strength training methods. In B. Jonsson (Ed.), *Biomechanics X-B* (pp. 615-620). Champaign, IL: Human Kinetics.

Schmidtbleicher, D. (1992). Training for power events. In P.V. Komi (Ed.), *Strength and Power in Sport* (pp. 381-395). Oxford: Blackwell Scientific Publications.

Sharkey, B.J. (1975). *Physiology and Fitness Activity.* New York: Harper & Row.

Shaver, L.G. (1981). *Essentials of Exercise Physiology.* Minneapolis: Burgess.

Silvester, L.J., Stiggins, C., McGown, C. & Bryce, G.R. (1982). The effect of variable resistance and free-weight training programs on strength and vertical jump. *National Strength and Conditioning Association Journal, 3* (6), 30-33.

Smith, M.J., & Melton, P. (1981). Isokinetic versus isotonic variable resistance training. *American Journal of Sports Medicine, 9* (4), 275-279.

Stadler, L.V., Stubbs, N.B. & Vukovich, M.D. (1997). A comparison of a 2-day and 3-day per week resistance training program on strength gains in older adults. *Medicine and Science in Sports and Exercise, 29,* 254.

Starkey, D.B., Pollock M.L., Ishida, Y., Welsch, M.A., Brechue, W.F., Graves, J.E. & Feigenbaum, M.S. (1996). Effect of resistance training volume on strength and muscle thickness. *Medicine and Science in Sports and Exercise, 28* (10), 1311-1320.

Staron, R.S., Karapondo, D.L., Kraemer, W.J., Fry, A.C., Gordon, S.E., Falkel, J.E., Hagerman, F.C. & Hikida, R.S. (1994). Skeletal muscle adaptations during early phase of heavy-resistance training in men and women. *Journal of Applied Physiology, 76* (3), 1247-1255.

Staron, R.S., Murray, T.E., Gilders, R.M., Hagerman, F.C., Hikida, R.S. & Ragg, K. E. (2000). Influence of resistance training on serum lipid and lipoprotein concentrations in young men and women. *Journal of Strength and Conditioning Research, 14* (1), 37-44.

Stone, M.H. (1988). Implications for connective tissue and bone alterations resulting from resistance exercise training. *Medicine and Science in Sports and Exercise, 20* (5), 162-168.

Stone, W.J. & Coulter, S.P. (1994). Strength/endurance effects from three resistance training protocols with women. *Journal of Strength and Conditioning Research, 8* (4), 231-234.

Stone, M.H., Fleck, S.J., Triplett, N.T. & Kraemer, W.J. (1991). Health- and performance-related potential of resistance training. *Sports Medicine, 11* (4), 210-231.

Stone, M.H. & O'Bryant, H.S. (1987). *Weight Training: A Scientific Approach.* Minneapolis: Burgess.

Stone, M.H., O'Bryant, H., Garhammer, J., McMillan, J. & Rozenek, R. (1982). A theoretical model of strength training. *National Strength and Conditioning Association Journal, 4* (4), 36-39.

Stone, M.H., Potteiger, J.A., Peirce, K.C., Proulx, C.M., O'Bryant H.S., Johnson, R.L. & Stone, M.E. (2000). Comparison of the effects of three different weight-training programs on the one repetition maximum squat. *Journal of Strength and Conditioning Research, 14* (3), 332-337.

Stone, M.H. & Wilson, G. (1985). Resistive training and selected effects. *Medical Clinics of North America, 69* (1), 109-122.

Stowers, T., McMillan, J., Scala, D., Davis, V., Wilson, D. & Stone, M. (1983). The short-term effects of three different strength-power training methods. *National Strength and Conditioning Association Journal, 5* (3), 24-27.

Taylor, J.M., Thompson, H.S., Clarkson, P.M., Miles, M.P. & De Souza, M.J. (2000). Growth hormone response to an acute bout of resistance exercise in weight-trained and non-weight-trained women. *Journal of Strength and Conditioning Research, 14* (2), 220-227.

Terbizan, D.J. & Bartels, R.I. (1985). The effect of set-repetition combinations on strength gain in females age 18-35. *Medicine and Science in Sports and Exercise, 17*, 267.

Tesch, P. (1988). Skeletal muscle adaptations consequent to long-term heavy resistance exercise. *Medicine and Science in Sports and Exercise, 20* (5), 132-134.

Tesch, P. (1992). Short-term and long-term histochemical and biochemical adaptations in muscle. In P.V. Komi (Ed.), *Strength and Power in Sport* (pp. 239-248). Oxford: Blackwell Scientific Publications.

Tesch, P. (1992). *Target Bodybuilding*. Champaign, IL: Human Kinetics.

Treuth, M.S., Ryan, A.S., Pratley, R.E, Rubin, M.A., Miller, J.P., Nicklas, B.J., Sorkin, J., Harman, S.M., Goldberg, A.P. & Hurley, B.F. (1994). Effects of strength training on total and regional body composition in older men. *Journal of Applied Physiology, 77* (2), 614-620.

Vincent, K., De Hoyos, D., Garzarella, L., Hass, C., Nordman, M. & Pollock, M. (1998). Relationship between indices of knee extension strength before and after training. *Medicine and Science in Sports and Exercise, 30* (5), 163.

Wathen, D. (1994). Muscle balance. In T.R. Baechle (Ed.), *Essentials of Training and Conditioning* (pp. 424-430). Champaign, IL: Human Kinetics.

Weiss, L.W., Coney, H.D. & Clark, F.C. (1999). Differential functional adaptations to short-term low-, moderate-, and high- repetition weight training. *Journal of Strength and Conditioning Research, 13* (3), 236-241.

Welsch, M.A., Brechue, W.F., Pollock, M.L., Starkey, D.B. & Graves, J.B. (1994). Effect of reduced training volume on bilateral isometric knee/extension torque. *Medicine and Science in Sports and Exercise, 26* (suppl), S189.

Wenzel, R.R. & Perfetto, E.M. (1992). The effect of speed versus non-speed training in power development. *Journal of Applied Sports Science Research, 6* (2), 82-87.

Westcott, W.L. (1986). 4 key factors in building a strength program. *Scholastic Coach, 55,* 104-105, 123.

Westcott, W.L., Greenberger, K. & Milius, D. (1989). Strength training research: sets and repetitions. *Scholastic Coach, 58* (10), 98-100.

Wilmore, J.H. (1982). *Training for sport and activity: the physiological basis of the conditioning process* (2nd edition). Boston: Allyn and Bacon.

Wilmore, J.H. & Costill, D.L. (1994). Neuromuscular adaptations to resistance training. In J.H. Wilmore & D.L. Costill (Eds.), *Physiology of sport and exercise* (pp. 66-89). Champaign, IL: Human Kinetics.

Wilmore, J.H. & Costill, D.L. (1994). *Physiology of Exercise and Sport.* Champaign, IL: Human Kinetics.

Winnett, R.A. & Carpinelli, R.N. (2000). Examining the validity of exercise guidelines for the prevention of morbidity and all-cause mortality. *Annals of Behavioral Medicine, 22,* 237-245.

Withers, R.T. (1970). Effect of varied weight-training loads on the strength of university freshmen. *Research Quarterly, 41* (1), 110-114.

Wolfe, B.L., LeMura, L.M. & Cole, P.J. (2004). Quantitative analysis of single vs. multiple-set programs in resistance training. *Journal of Strength and Conditioning Research, 18* (1), 35-47.

Womack, C.J., Flohr, J.A., Weltman, A. & Gaesser, G. (2000). The effects of a short-term training program on the slow component of VO_2. *Journal of Strength and Conditioning Research, 14,* 50-53.

Zatsiorsky, V.M. (1995). *Science and Practice of Strength Training.* Champaign, IL: Human Kinetics.

Acknowledgements

I would like to thank everybody who helped to make this book possible. My thanks go to all colleagues and authors who are mentioned, quoted or referenced in this book. I especially thank Christina Teigland and illustrators Julia Suchoroschenko and Udo Buffler. Last but not least I would like to thank my students and readers for giving me feedback on their success with High Intensity Training.

About the author

Jürgen Giessing is a professor of sports science at the University of Koblenz-Landau in Germany and teaches training science and sports medicine at the Landau campus. His main field of research is the process of training, physiological adaptation to training and factors that are relevant for muscle building. With two or three workouts per week, each lasting between 30 and 50 minutes, he keeps his body fat level between six and eight percent all year round.

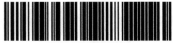

Made in the USA
Middletown, DE
08 December 2018